THE TECHNIQUES OF LADIES' HAIRDRESSING OF THE 19TH CENTURY

A Compilation of Original 19th Century Sources
by Mark Campbell and Mons. A. Mallemont

edited by
Jules & Kaethe Kliot

LACIS
PUBLICATIONS
Berkeley, CA 94703

The work of this book is taken, essentially unabridged, from two very important manuals of this period:

SELF-INSTRUCTOR IN THE ART OF HAIR WORK: DRESSING HAIR, MAKING CURLS, SWITCHES, BRAIDS AND HAIR JEWELRY OF EVERY DESCRIPTION by Mark Campbell published in 1875.

[*The section devoted to Hair Jewelry and the section 'Synopsis of Human Hair' has been reprinted separately by this publisher under the title THE ART OF HAIRWORK, HAIR BRAIDING AND JEWELRY OF SENTIMENT, Lacis Publications, 1989.*]

and

MANUAL OF LADIES' HAIRDRESSING FOR STUDENTS by Mons. A. Mallemont originally published in French, 1899

[*Original page numbers have been left intact as is the original table of contents.*]

The fashion plates illustrating the relation of hair to headwear and to the female silhouette are from the following contemporary magazines:

LA MODE ILLUSTREE, *1877*
GODEY'S FASHIONS, *1877*
GODEY'S FASHIONS, *1878*
PETERSON'S MAGAZINE, *1884*
YOUNG LADIES' JOURNAL, *Dec. 1887*
TOILETTES, *October 1893*
TOILETTES, *November 1894*
TOILETTES, *December 1894*
LA MODE DE PARIS, *January 1895*
TOILETTES, *February 1895*
LE COSTUME ROYAL, *December 1897*
ELITE STYLES, *November 1898*

LACIS
PUBLICATIONS
3163 Adeline Street, Berkeley, CA 94703

ISBN 0-916896-71-4

LADIES' HAIRDRESSING
OF THE 19TH CENTURY

There are few periods in human history when the hair covering of the head was not at the forefront of fashion. Whether in the form of wigs made from the finest imported hair, hair appendages, or simply using ones natural assets, the design of coiffures would range from short unruly curls to the absurd allegorical coiffures of the court of Louis XIV to the very stylized and manicured forms so popular in our current age.

The early part of the 19th century was a reprieve from the fanciful hair fashions of the previous century. Fashions so elementary that the professional hairdresser was unnecessary...a simple clipped on chignon or turban being the mode. By the 1830's with the influence of the industrial revolution, unsuccessful attempts were made for dramatic change. Metal forms, wire mesh loops and high combs were to challenge the closely-cropped cut. Along with the spirit of the Victorian age, the submissive woman, prevailed. Hairstyles were to remain tight to the head, highly stylized, and if not covered by the pervasive bonnet, designed as if it should be.

By the 1870's the bonnet was replaced by the small hat. Perched on top of the head it called for an abundance of hair and in many cases it was indistinguishable from the coiffure which was often embellished with similar feathers, beads and other appendages. It is the exuberance of this period, which led to a whole new vocabulary of hair styling, that is the focus of this book. The chignon or length of hair which could be knotted in a prescribed fashion, coiled or rolled in curls were the vogue. Initially these were imported hairpieces, later as health problems relating to unhygenic hair pieces were reported, the growing of long tresses became quite common, with natural hair left to grow to one's knees. By the 1880s the use of hot irons to wave and curl the hair did much to influence the later styles of this period.

Hair, of course, was only part of the total image. The context of these styles can not be ignored as hair styles and costume went hand-in-hand. The striking style changes during the last decades of the 19th c. are presented in a collection of images from some of the many fashion magazines of the period. While the hat was most directly related to the hair style, it was the overall silhouette which had to be satisfied. In the 1880's the exaggerated bustle was the vogue. The vertical hair/hat was a natural to emphasize this awkward silhouette. During the early 1890's the focus was on the shoulders, to which all other parts of the body were designed to emphasize. The waist and head were minimized while famed leg-o-mutton sleeves reached huge proportions. By the end of the decade, emphasis was directed to the head with hair styles and hats emphasized by size and elaborate design, the leg-o-mutton sleeve virtually disappearing.

CONTENTS

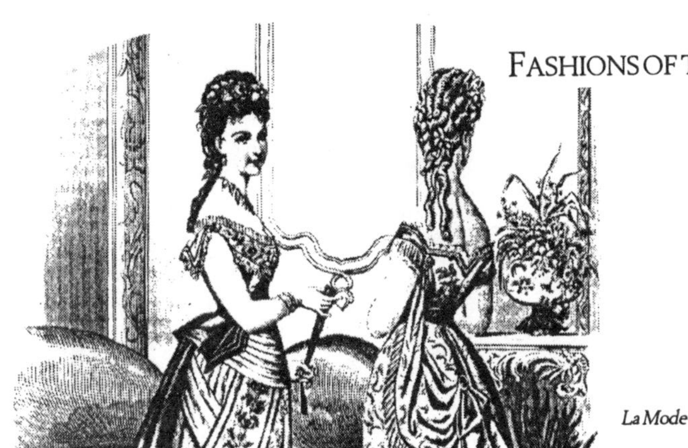

La Mode Illustree, 1877

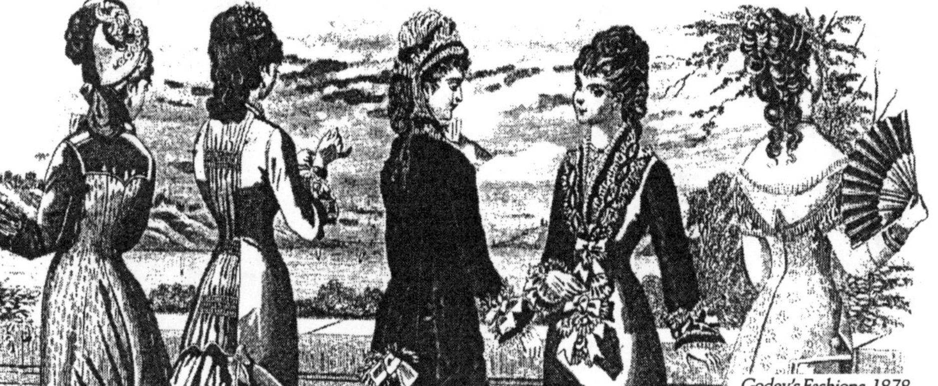

Godey's Fashions, 1878

Godey's Fashions, 1877

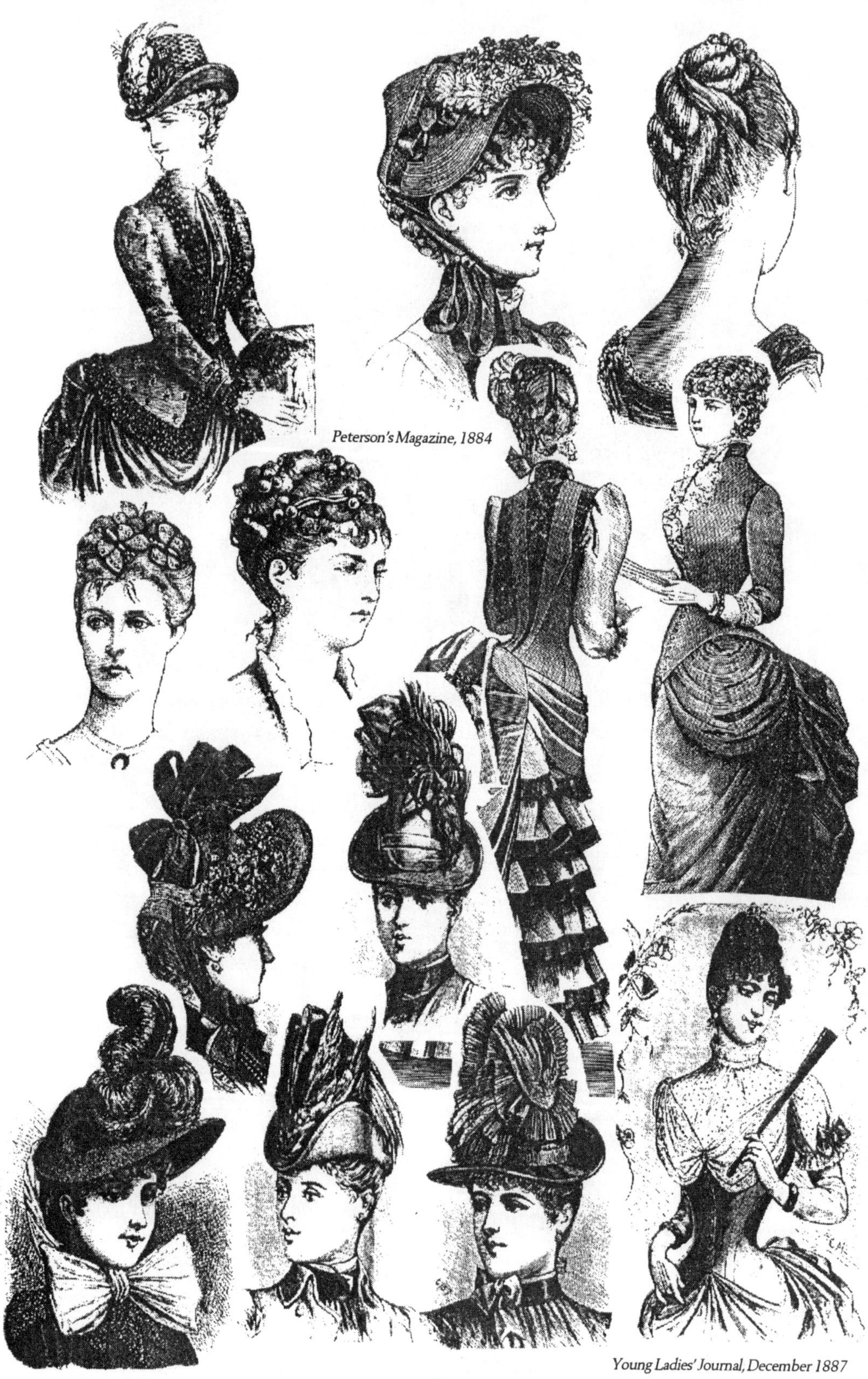

Peterson's Magazine, 1884

Young Ladies' Journal, December 1887

Weaving Hair for Switchs.

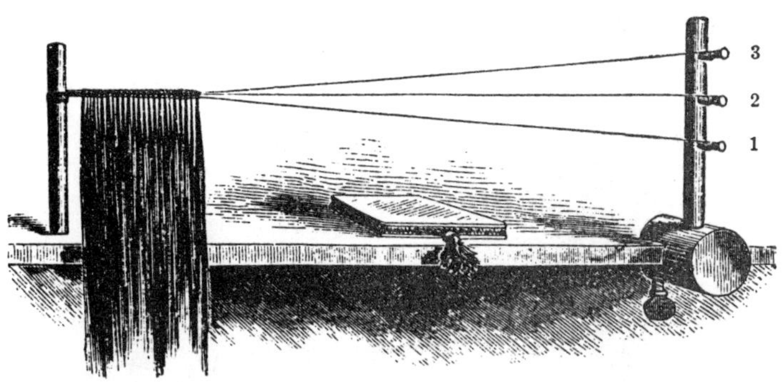

The above cut represents the apparatus used for weaving hair into Switches, Curls, Wigs, etc. It is a very simple arrangement, and can be easily constructed. Provide two straight sticks, about twelve inches long, and in one of them bore three small holes, two inches apart, in which to place as many thumb-screws, to be used for tightening or loosening the cords; in the other, have a single wooden pin or nail, to fasten the cords to. Place the sticks in a firm, upright position, about three feet apart, either by boring holes through a table, or by using mortised blocks, such as is plainly shown in cut, at the right end. After placing them in position, put on three cords, as shown in diagram, numbered 1, 2 and 3. For this weft use linen thread, at Nos. 1, 2 and 3.

In commencing to weave, place the hair between two cards, as shown in diagram, and draw out with the right hand, between the thumb and fore-finger, the quantity of hair required for the size of the weft; then change it into the left hand, and place it up to the threads, Nos. 1, 2 and 3, as shown in diagram; lay the strand over No. 1, under No. 2, over No. 3, around under No. 3, over Nos. 2 and 1, around under Nos. 1 and 2, over No. 3, around under Nos. 3 and 2, and over No. 1. Then push the strands together, as in cut.

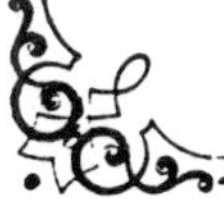

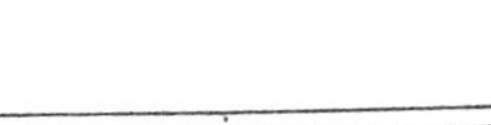

Sewing Switches.

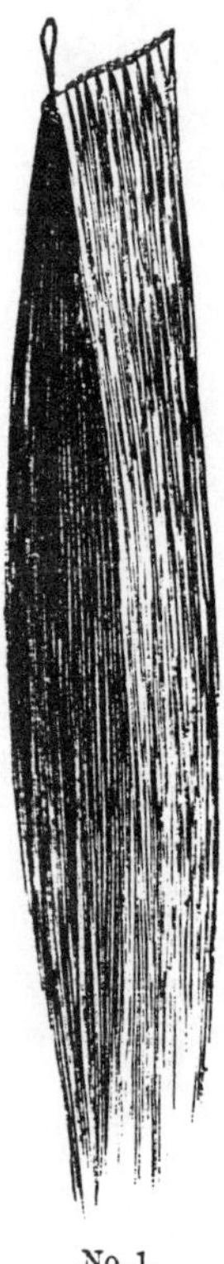

No. 1.

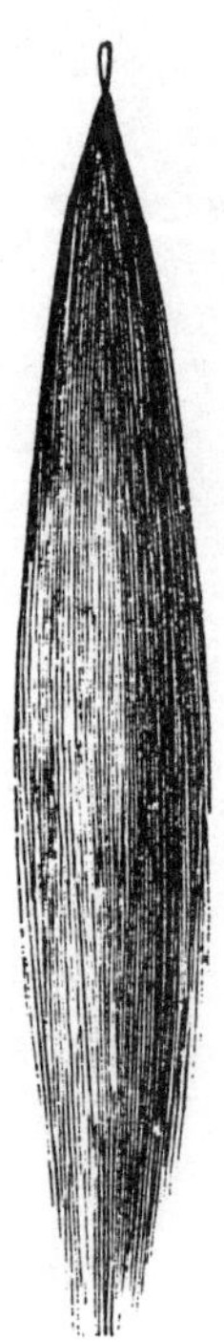

No. 2.

The No. 1 of the above cuts represents the winding and sewing of the switch after it is woven.   For sewing a switch on points, after weaving, take Berlin cord, about one-sixteenth of an inch thick, and tie a solid knot at the end, and sew the end of the weft to the knotted end of the cord; then wind the weft around the cord, as shown in cut, the length of point desired, turning the end of the cord over to form a loop.   Cut the weft according to the number of points desired in the switch.   Cut No. 2 shows the switch all complete.

Weaving Hair for Curls.

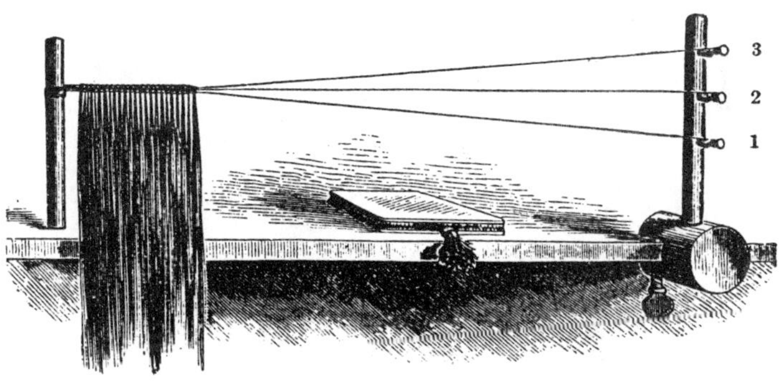

In commencing to weave, place the hair between two cards, or stiff brushes, as shown in diagram, pressing them tight together, so that in drawing out it is perfectly free from tangles; draw out with the right hand, between the thumb and fore-finger, the quantity of hair required for the size of the weft; then change it into the left hand, and lift it up to the No. 1 cord, as shown in diagram; lay the strand over No. 1, under No. 2, over No. 3, around under No. 3, over Nos. 2 and 1, around under Nos. 1 and 2, over No. 3, around under No. 3, over No. 2, and under No. 1. Then push the strands together, as shown in diagram. For this weft use fine, strong linen thread.

Making and Preparing Curls.

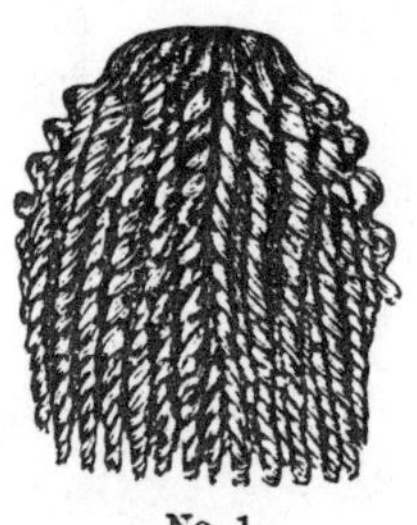

No. 1.

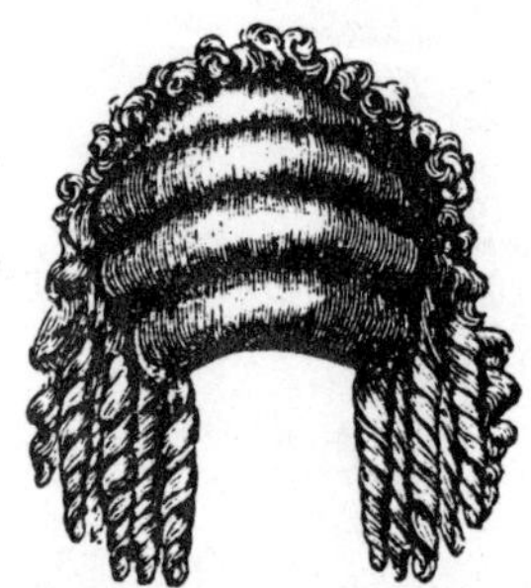

No. 2.

After weaving, according to directions on page 241, take a piece of ribbon an inch wide, the same color of hair, and as long as you wish the curls to be in width, and sew the weft to it back and forth. After that is done, pipe them, which is done in this manner: Dampen the hair, comb each curl out straight, and wind it tightly on a rattan stick about four inches long, having each curl on a separate stick, and commencing to wind at the tip end, tying them firmly to keep in place. Then boil in water for thirty minutes, and place in an oven as hot as they will bear without burning, until quite dry. When dry and perfectly cool, take them off the sticks, and smooth over a curling iron, the size you wish the curls. Side curls and frizzes should be prepared the same way.

Cut No. 2 represents a set of Curls and Puffs. For explanations of Puffs, see page 245.

Weaving Hair for Wigs.

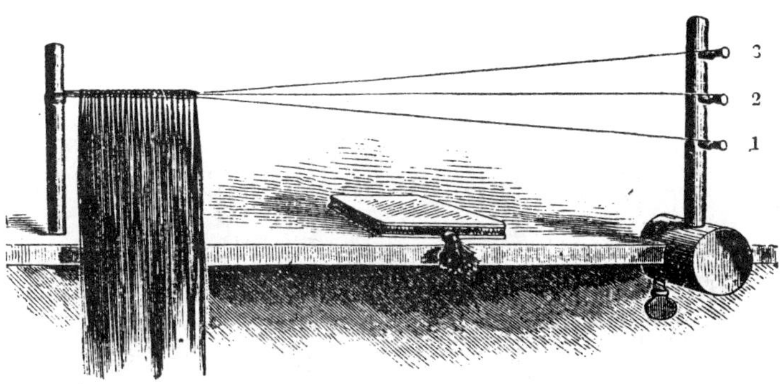

In commencing to weave, place the hair between two cards, or stiff brushes, as shown in diagram, pressing them tight together, so that in drawing out, it is perfectly free from tangles; draw out with the right hand, between the thumb and fore-finger, the quantity of hair required for the size of the weft; then change it into the left hand, and lift it up to the No. 1 cord, as shown in diagram; lay the strand over No. 1, under No. 2, over No. 3, around under No. 3, over Nos. 2 and 1, around under Nos. 1 and 2, over No. 3, around under No. 3, over Nos. 2 and 1, around under Nos. 1 and 2, over No. 3, around under Nos. 3 and 2, and over No. 1. Then push the strands together, as shown in diagram. For this weft use sewing silk.

WEAVING HAIR FOR WATERFALLS AND BOWS.

Prepare the same as above, and place the strand under No. 1, over Nos. 2 and 3, around under Nos. 3 and 2, over No. 1, around under Nos. 1 and 2, over No. 3, around under No. 3, and over Nos. 2 and 1. Aside from these changes, follow directions given above.

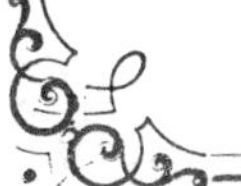
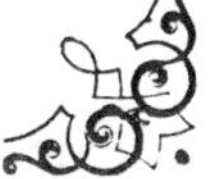

Making Waterfalls and Bows.

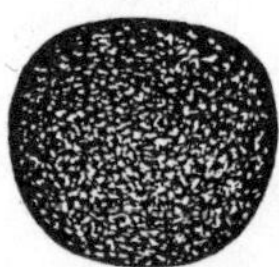

No. 1.

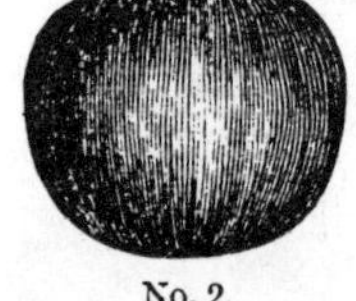

No. 2.

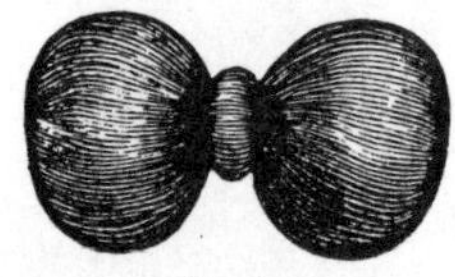

No. 3.

In making a Chignon, you have first to make the cushion. Take the combings or waste hair, which is of no other use, and place it between the cards or stiff brushes, the same as for weaving. Use the weaving apparatus, with two piping cords, instead of three small ones, and wind the hair all up, by passing over, between and under the cords. Boil and dry it, and then pull out the cord, which leaves it all crimped, ready to weave, according to directions on page 239. Then sew it on a cord, the same as a switch, and form it in any shape you desire, for a Waterfall, Bow or Puffs. This completes the cushion. Then weave the long hair for the covering, according to directions on page 243, and sew it to the top end of the cushion; comb it out smooth, cover the cushion, and tie a cord around it immediately at the bottom; then bring up the end of the hair, and pin it to the inside. Cut No. 1 is intended to represent the cushion, and No. 2 the complete Waterfall.

Cut No. 3 represents the Bow, which is made in the same manner, by using two small cushions, like cut No. 1, and placing between them a strand of smooth or braided hair.

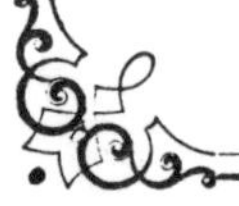

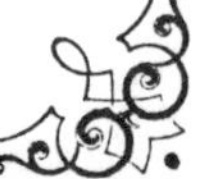

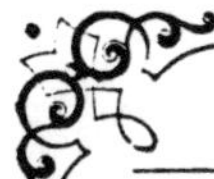

Making Puffs and Coils.

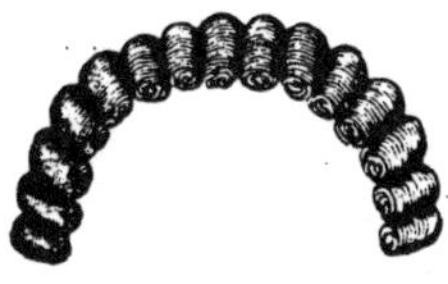

No. 1.

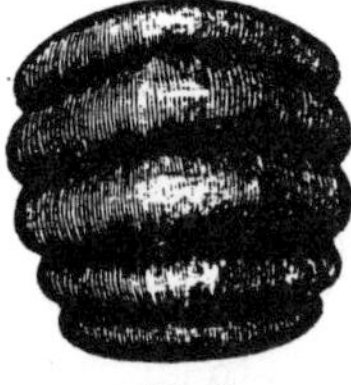

No. 2.

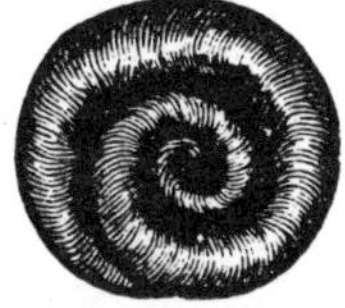

No. 3.

To make Puffs for front of head, from false hair, similar to cut No. 1, weave hair from eight to twelve inches long, according to directions on page 241; then take a ribbon, about one and a half inches wide, any length required, and tack it on a wig block, or straight piece of board, and sew the weft crosswise a quarter of an inch apart, till the ribbon is entirely covered; then divide it off in as many puffs as desired, comb each out straight, and wind it over the two fore-fingers, close up to ribbon, and put in a hair-pin to retain it.

To make Puffs for back of head, cut No. 2, prepare the same way; make the foundation the shape and size you wish the puffs, and sew it on the same way you want the puffs to run. The puffs may be made over a cushion, formed of crimped hair the shape wanted, and wound over that instead of the fingers. Ladies not wearing false hair, can have their own hair dressed by following the above directions.

Cut No. 3 represents a coil, which is made from a switch, and wound over a long roll of crimped hair. They are much nicer, but more expensive, by being made altogether from a switch, as that can be twisted into a rope or braided, before coiling.

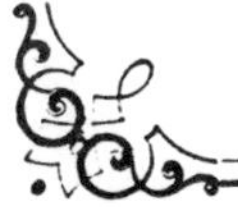

Explanations on Hair Dressing.

I herewith present, on the following pages, a number of engravings illustrative of a few of the many styles of Hair Dressing, accompanied with explanatory remarks as to their execution. They are the latest and most fasionable European and American styles, and will prove indispensable to every lady's toilet, as, from the explanations, they will be able, with very little practice, to dress their own hair in any desired style; and when any new style is inaugurated, after studying and practicing the directions given with each illustration, they will find it an easy matter to arrange it accordingly.

Any one learning Hair Dressing, should acquire perfectly the execution of the first pattern—the Promenade Head-Dress—as that is very easily arranged, and when you have once executed it in a perfect manner, the others will prove comparatively easy.

The manner of dressing the hair at the present day calls for much attention, and many inquiries are addressed us on the subject. It is plain, however, that what would correspond with the complexion and physiognomy of one, would certainly have a distasteful appearance on another; consequently, in answering inquiries, I can do nothing more than give the different styles worn. Before giving my illustrations on Hair Dressing, I have given instructions how to weave hair for chignons, curls, switches, etc., and how to put them in shape, and with the directions given with each illustration on Hair Dressing, it will certainly be an easy task to arrange the hair in any style that is now or may be in fashion.

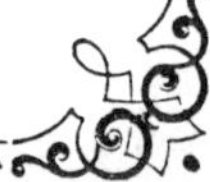

Hair Dressing.

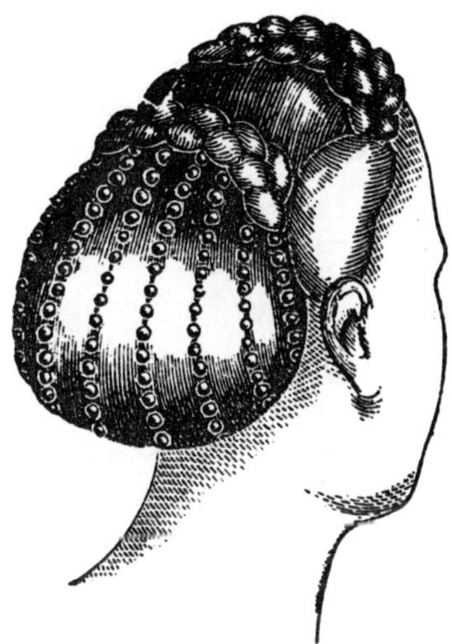

PROMENADE HEAD-DRESS.

Our first cut represents the Promenade Head-Dress, but is worn as frequently in the drawing-room, and even at public and private assemblies—in fact, a common and very pretty style.

EXPLANATION: Comb the front hair between the temples straight back, over a cushion of crimped hair, forming a chignon; then make two braids of two small switches, and place one of them over the top of the chignon, and the other across the forehead, forming a diadem, turning the ends under; then comb the hair from temples over the braids, and put back under the chignon, and fasten. Place a net of pearl or gilt beads over the chignon, as in cut. You can use false hair for covering cushion, if desired.

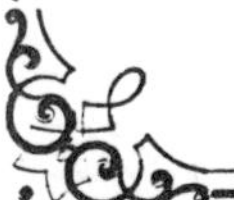

Hair Dressing.

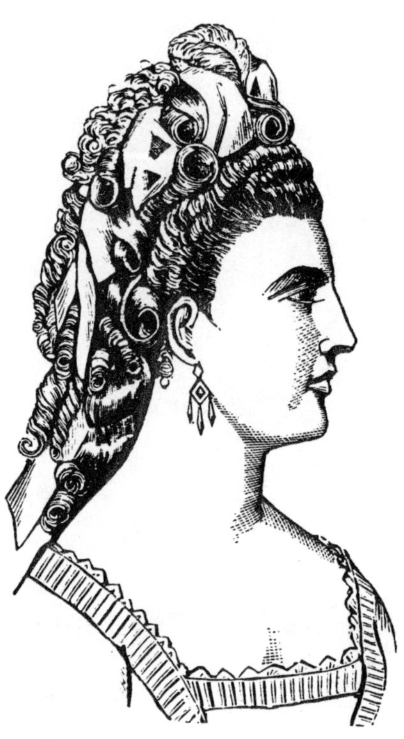

RECEPTION HEAD-DRESS.

This Head-Dress is a most charming composition, and entirely new. It is adapted either for a brown or fair complexion, to be worn at grand dinners or receptions. Ornamented with pearl or gilt, it is in good taste for evening parties.

EXPLANATION: Comb the hair all back; then crimp and curl the ends, or use false curls; form a chignon of curls and puffs at the back; make a wreath of ribbons, long curls and feather. Trim with roses and ribbons, or to suit dress.

Hair Dressing,

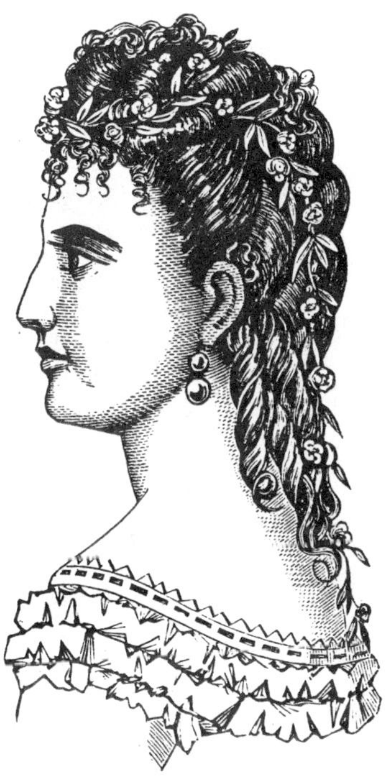

SOIREE OR EVENING HEAD-DRESS.

This cut illustrates the Soiree or Evening Head-Dress. It is a very unique and modern style, suited for almost any complexion, and very easily executed

EXPLANATION: Comb the hair back off the face, and curl the ends on the neck, or use a set of false curls; puff the hair from the forehead to the hollow of the neck, and put a set of short curls or frizes across the temples; then put flowers or ribbons between the puffs, to suit the dress or your taste. You may use a fancy back comb, or gilt or jet bands, but trim to suit dress.

Hair Dressing.

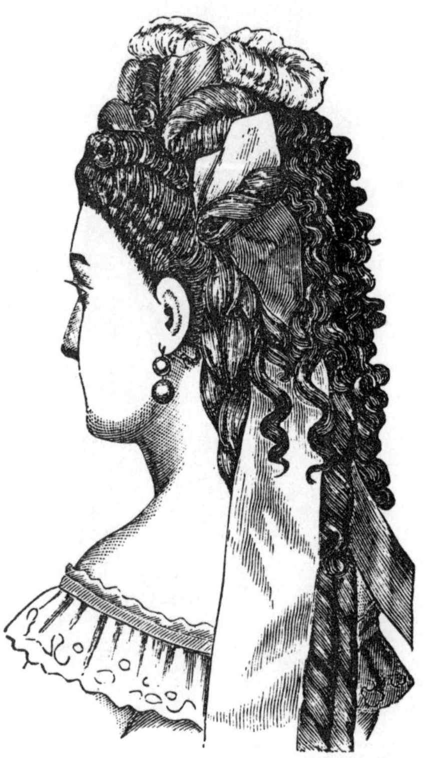

GRAND EVENING PARTY HEAD-DRESS.

A very graceful Head-Dress, of a bold style, suited for a young lady of brown or fair complexion, and is in good taste to be worn at the theatre or grand evening parties.

EXPLANATION: Comb the hair all back off the face; crimp, and let all fall back; curl some of the ends, or put some long curls at the back, and put a false braid to hang down from the back of the left ear; make three or four loose puffs on top of the forehead; then trim the hair with ribbons and feathers, as shown in the cut.

Hair Dressing.

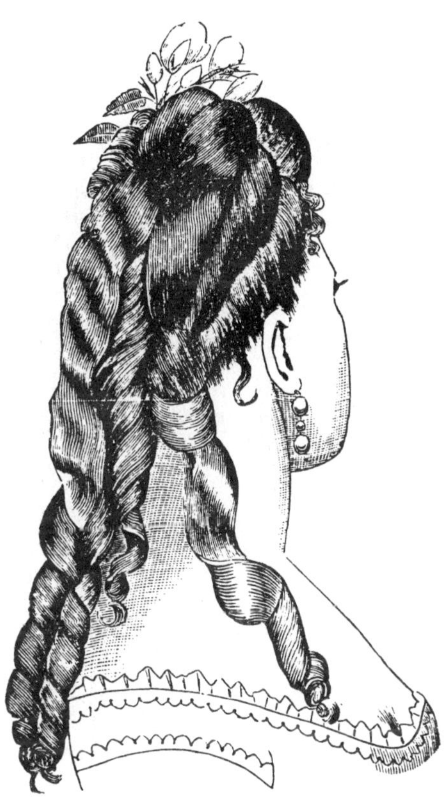

PROMENADE HEAD-DRESS.

A charming Head-Dress, entirely new, and perfectly suiting a fair complexion. It may serve for the theatre or evening parties. When powered, it is very suitable for a brown or brunette.

EXPLANATION: Comb the hair all up, and fringe the short all round the face; make two long puffs over rats at each side, and a large, loose butterfly bow on top of the head, leaving long ends; crimp and curl the ends, as shown in the cut, with a bunch of roses at one side of the bow. This style can be worn with a comb.

Hair Dressing.

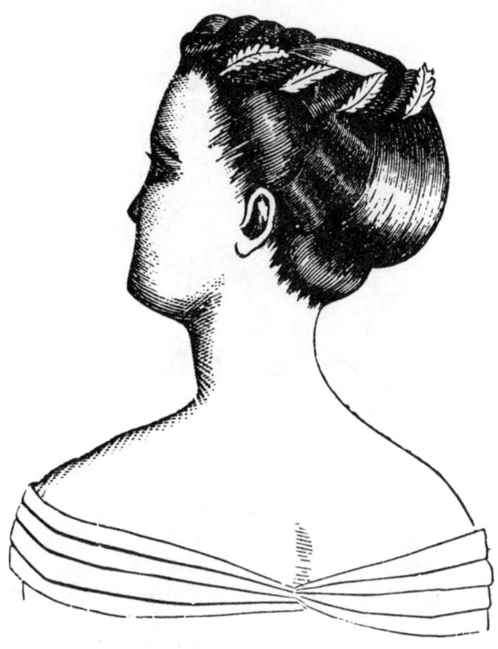

PARISIAN HEAD-DRESS.

This Head-Dress, both bold and graceful, is suitable for any complexion or age, when the physiognomy allows it.

EXPLANATION: Comb back the hair from the forehead between the temples, make a large puff on the temples, and three puffs above each ear. Place a cushion at the back of head, and comb the hair over it, forming a chignon; then place a diadem plait or twist, made from a large switch, round on the top of head, trimmed with leaves or ribbon, as shown in cut.

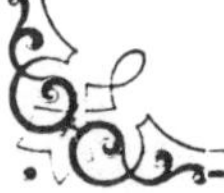
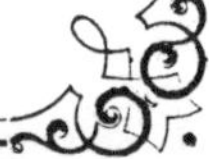

Hair Dressing.

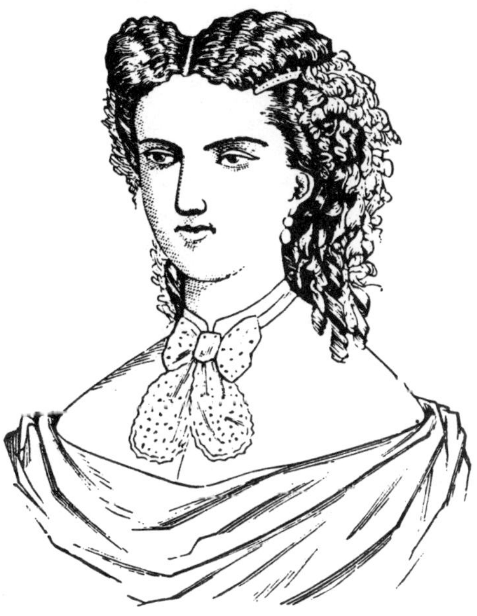

THE APOLLO HEAD-DRESS.

This Head-Dress is one of the most graceful styles. It was worn in the time of Louis XIV., and well agrees with the fashion of the present day. With some modifications, it is suited to every complexion.

EXPLANATION: Crimp the front hair, and raise it over the temples with a puff comb. Comb back the hair just above the ears, and friz the ends, and curl the back hair in large flowing curls, as shown in the cut,

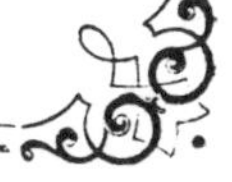

Hair Dressing.

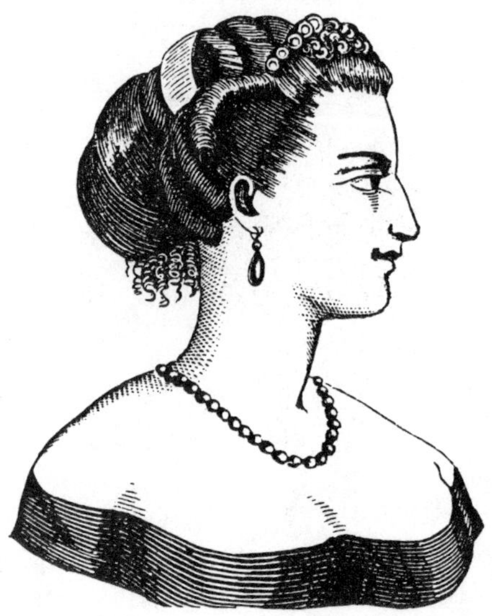

THE MODERN HEAD-DRESS.

A Head-Dress of elegant composition, coming down from antiquity, suitable for a young and pretty woman, and perfectly agreeing with a fair complexion.

EXPLANATION: Part the hair from temple to temple, one inch from front, comb it up on the forehead, and curl the ends in small snap curls; then comb the hair back from the temples, and form a loose puff. Make three partings across the head, and form a puff of each. Of the back hair, make a braided or plaited chignon, with a few friz curls underneath; then make two puffs back of the ear, as shown in cut. Wear a fancy comb or band over the top of chignon.

Hair Dressing.

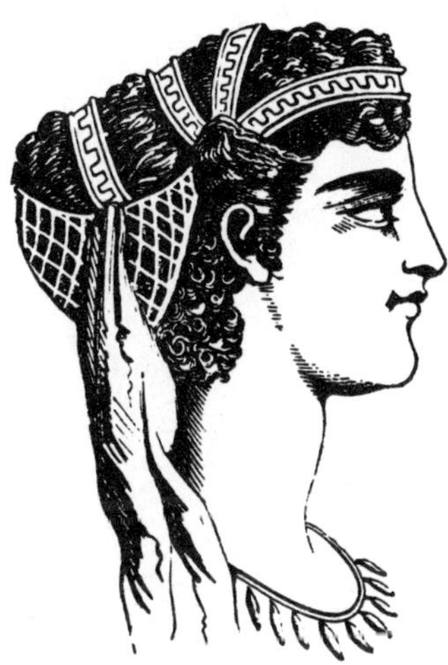

EVENING PROMENADE HEAD-DRESS.

A Head-Dress of extraordinary simplicity, and of a most genteel kind, becoming a dark complexion. It may be adapted for the opera by changing the trimming.

EXPLANATION: First crimp all the hair, then place a cushion high up under the hair at the back, forming a chignon, and friz the ends of the hair from ear to ear under the chignon. Tuck the hair high up on the forehead, place bands of ribbon over the head with a net at the back, and bring the hair above the ear up, and fasten to the ribbon. Pin a ribbon streamer to the net, as in cut.

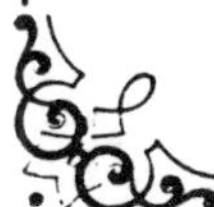

Hair Dressing.

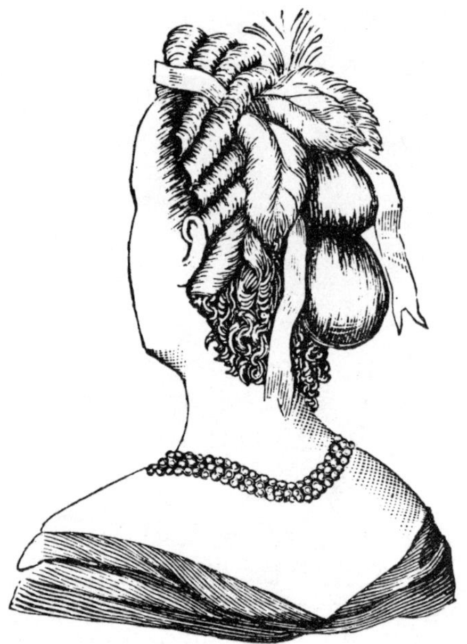

THE SHEPHERDESS HEAD-DRESS.

An elegant Head-Dress, and was worn in the time of Louis XVI., for balls and evening parties, or as a disguise when powdered.

EXPLANATION: Separate the hair across the head from ear to ear, three inches from front, and roll it in puffs according to directions on page 247. Do up the back hair in a double chignon, either with your own or false hair; add a set of false curls underneath the chignon, extending from ear to ear. Trim to suit dress with leaves, flowers and ribbon, as shown in illustration.

Hair Dressing.

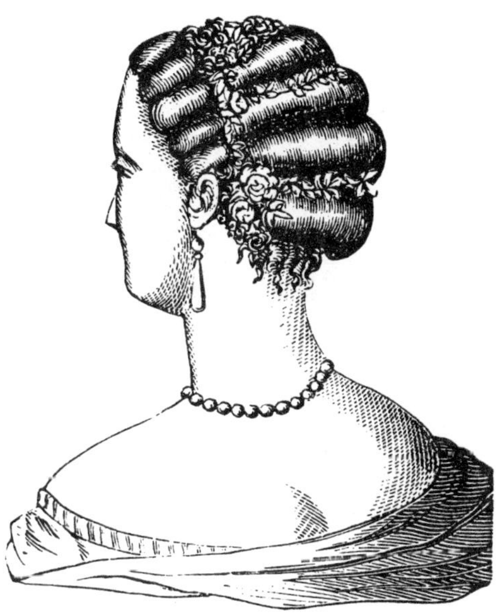

COURT HEAD-DRESS.

A rich Head-Dress, having a great stamp of distinction, and for that reason will be adapted for a Court Head-Dress, or grand evening parties.

EXPLANATION: Make a parting over the head from ear to ear, two inches from front, and form a row of nine small puffs over the forehead. Comb the remaining hair back, and divide into four partings around the head, and form each parting in a large puff, as in cut. Add a few small friz curls and orange blossoms between the puffs. For reference, see page 247.

Hair Dressing.

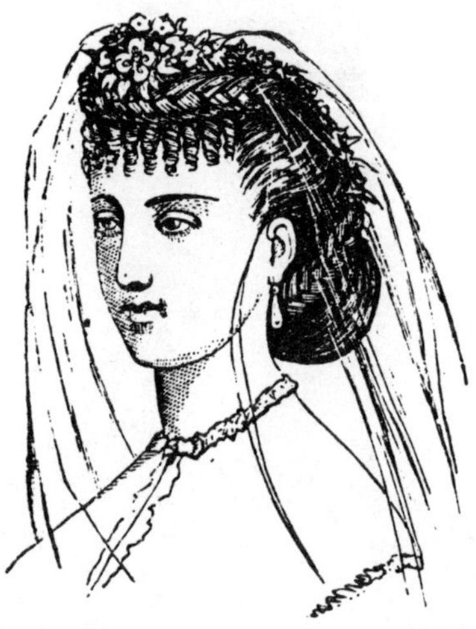

YOUNG BRIDE'S HEAD-DRESS.

An exquisite Head-Dress, of a very graceful style, and well agreeing with a fair or brown complexion, to be worn by a young bride, or at grand assemblies.

EXPLANATION: Comb the hair back and place a set of small loose curls across the forehead; place a diadem plait over the top of the curls, and comb the hair off the temples over the ends of the plait, and form a chignon or bow of the back hair, and place a three-strand braid around the chignon, made either from the ends of hair from the temple or a switch. Add a crown of white blossoms and a veil, as shown in the engraving. If not for a bride, trim to match dress.

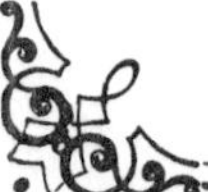

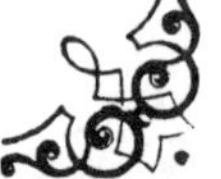

Hair Dressing.

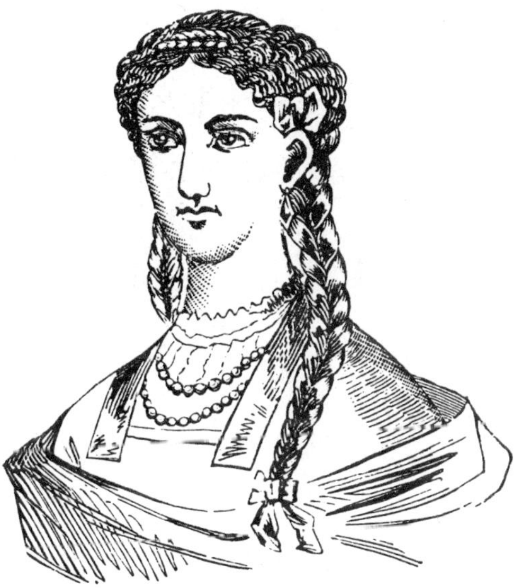

NEAPOLITAN HEAD-DRESS.

An exquisite Head-Dress, of exceedingly graceful and modern style, agreeing with nearly every complexion; may be worn at a promenade, or at small parties.

EXPLANATION: Part the hair from front to crown, and from ear to ear: crimp the front, and braid the ends in a three-strand braid, and trim the ends with ribbon. Either braid or twist the back hair, and form into a coil. Place a small plait across the forehead, as shown in the engraving. Deck the hair with flowers or beads, to suit the occasion.

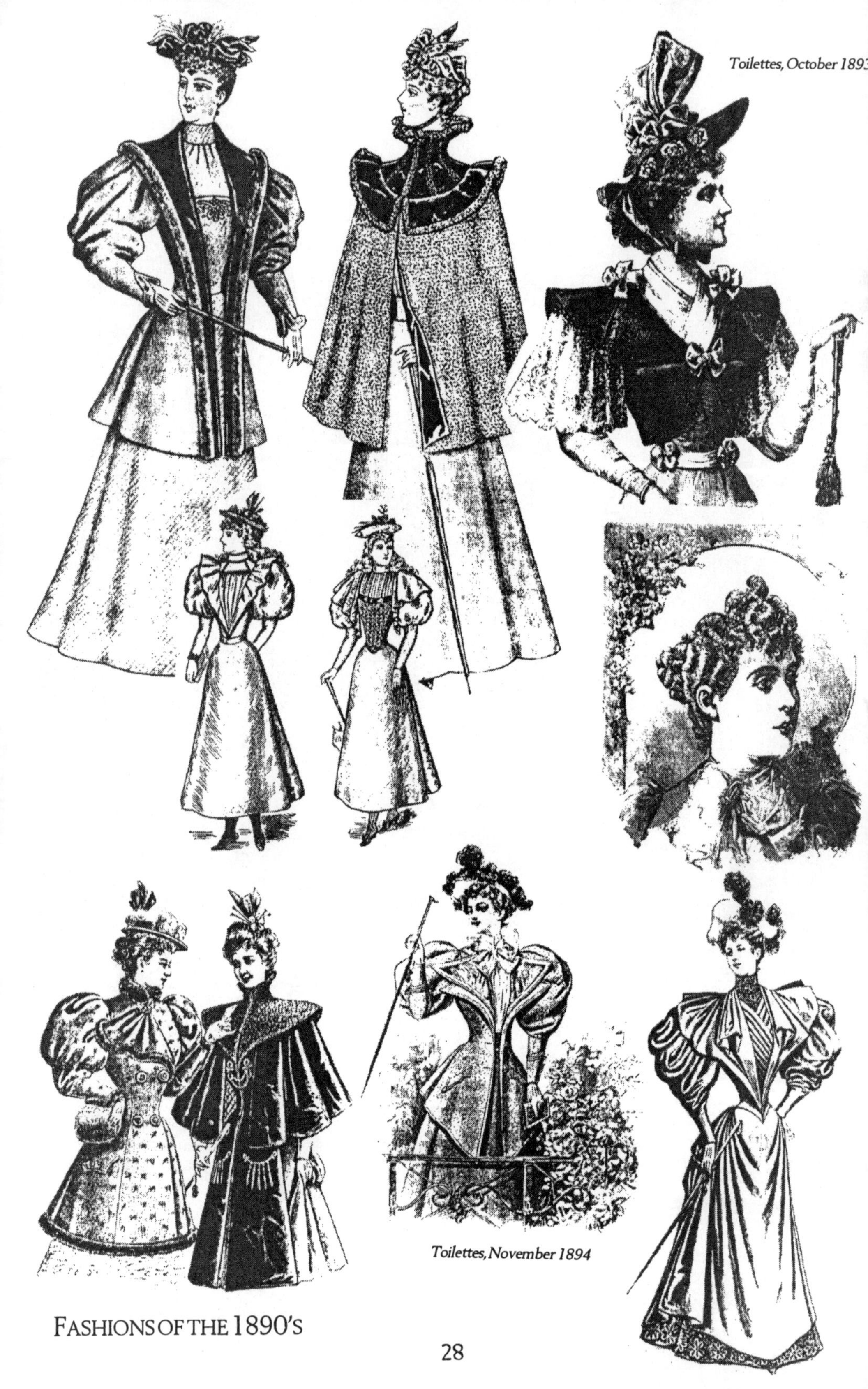

FASHIONS OF THE 1890's

28

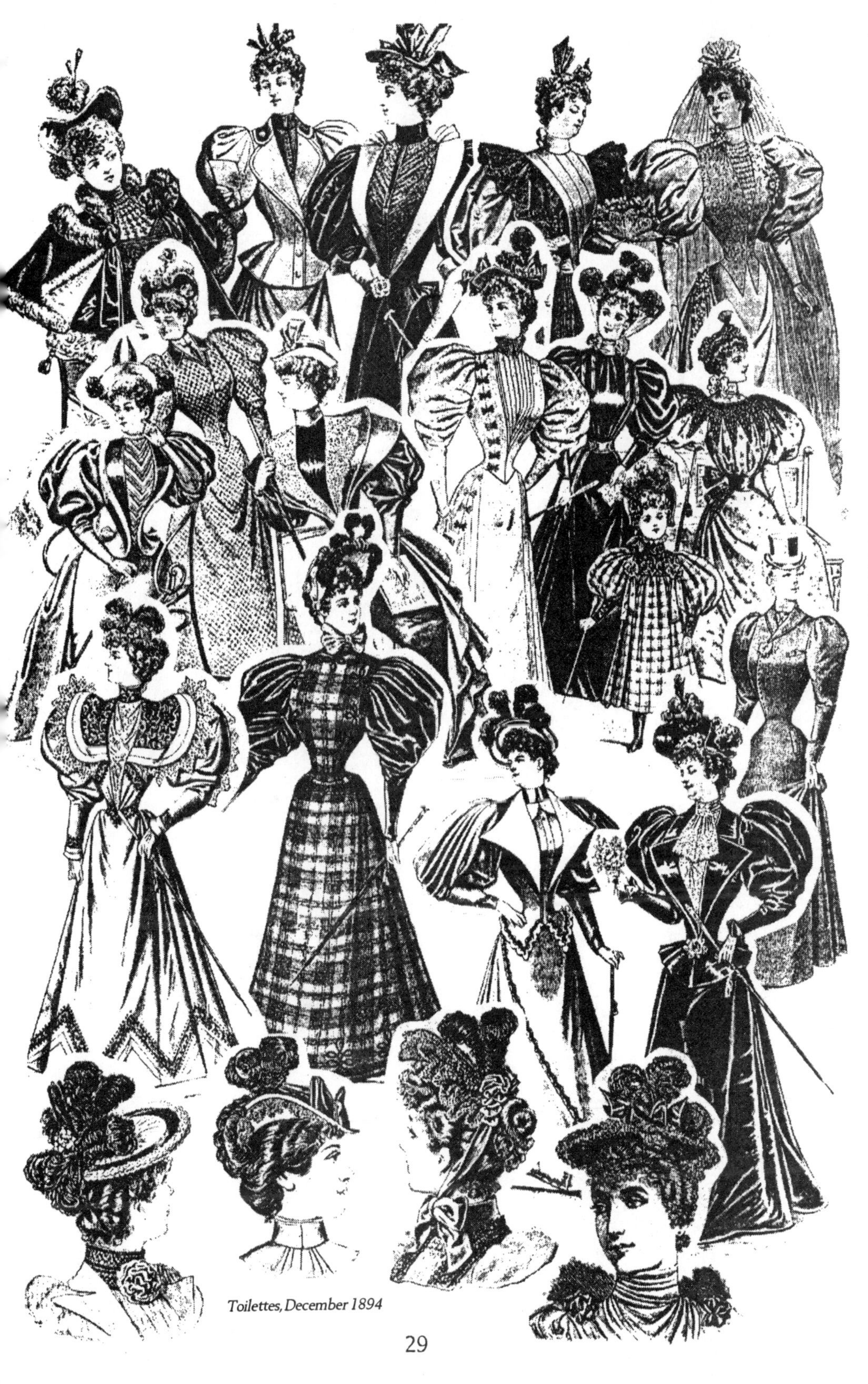

Toilettes, December 1894

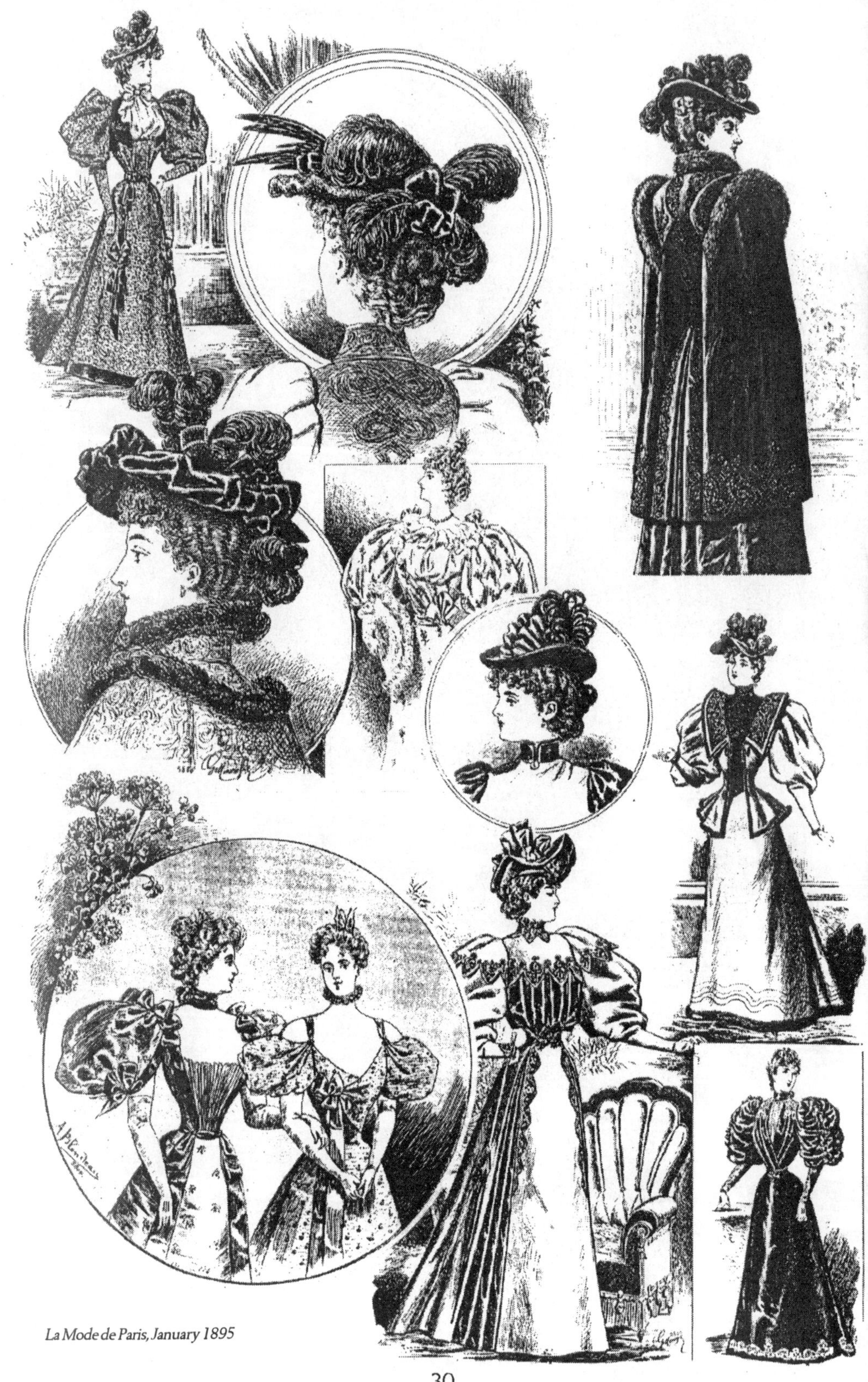

La Mode de Paris, January 1895

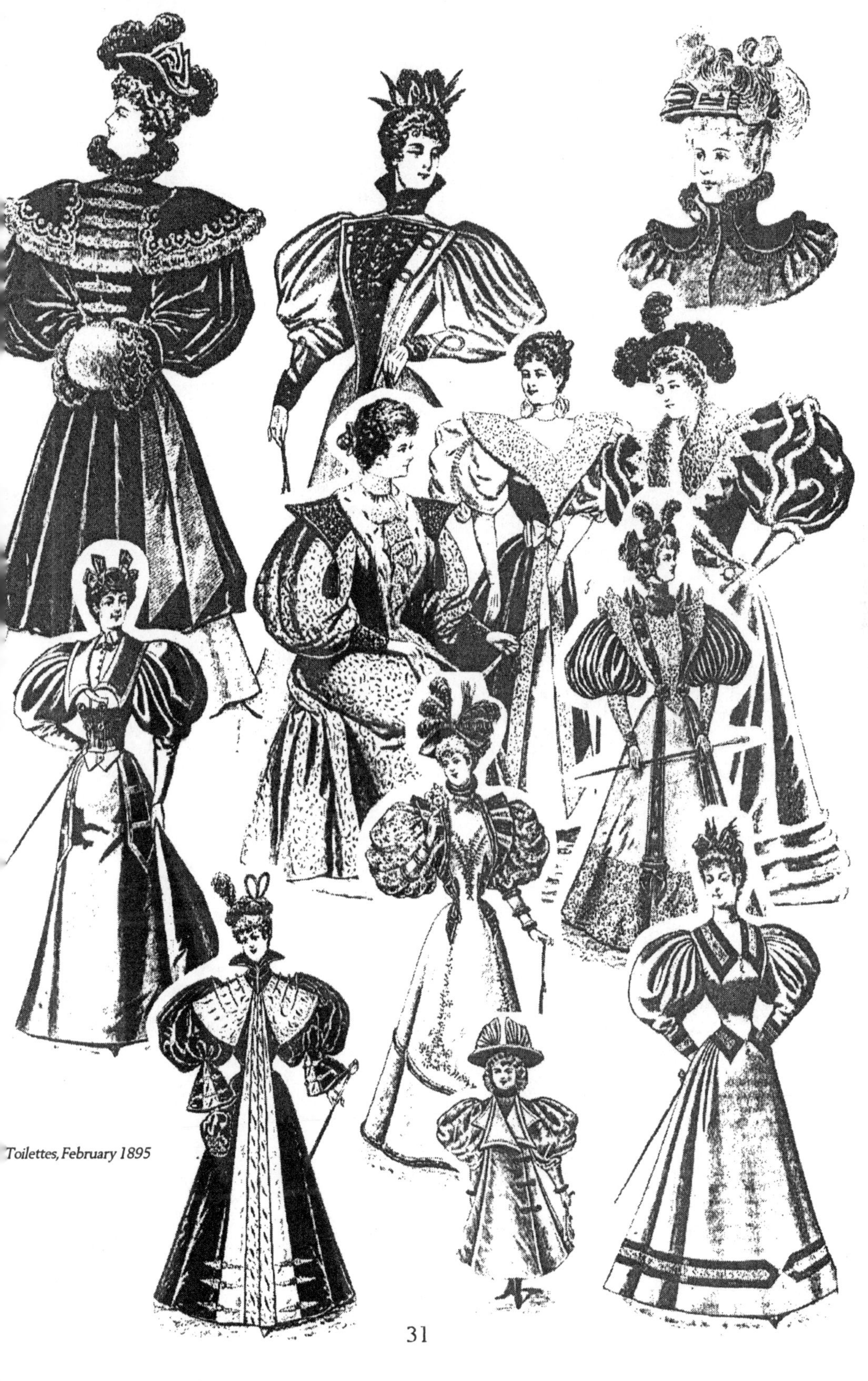

Toilettes, February 1895

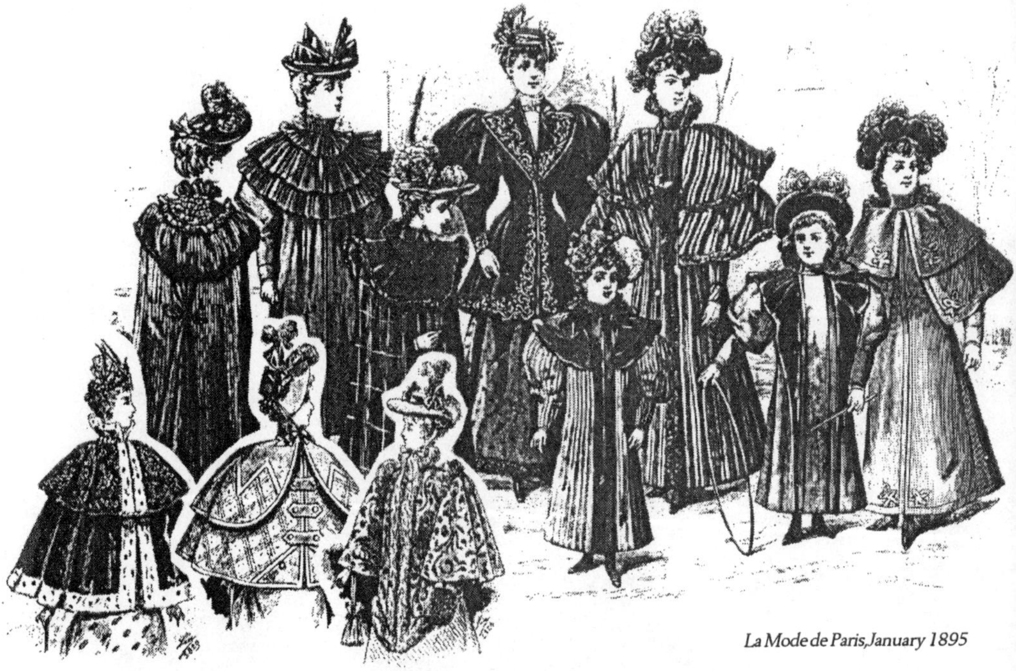

La Mode de Paris, January 1895

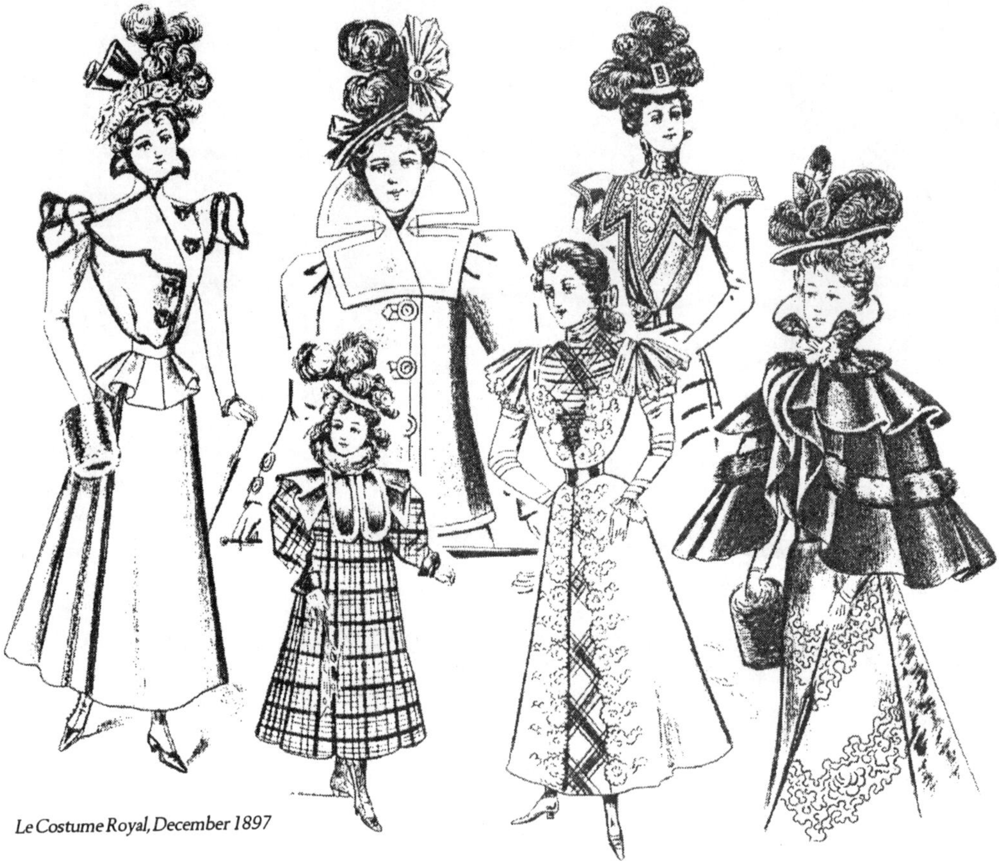

Le Costume Royal, December 1897

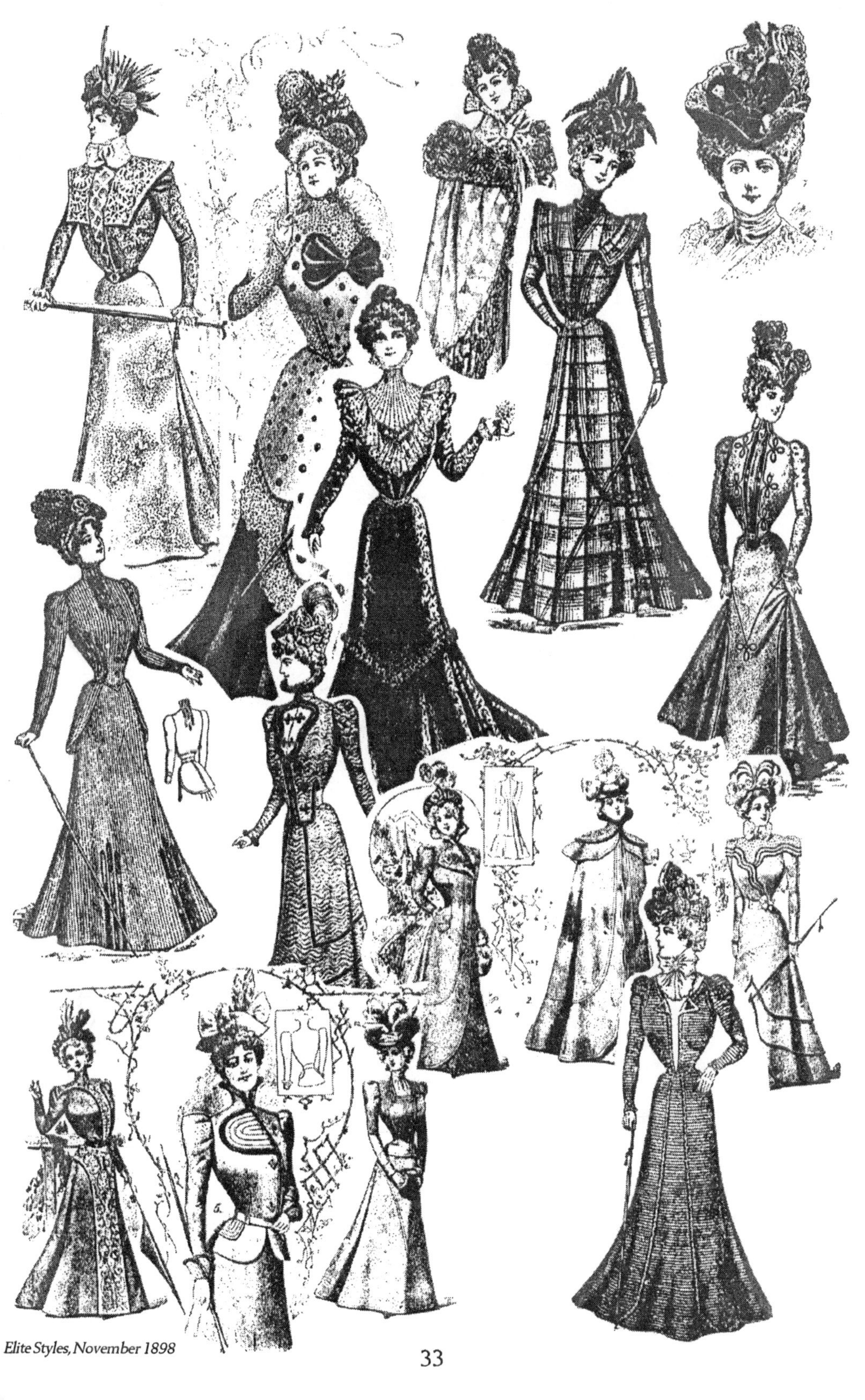

MANUAL

OF

LADIES' HAIRDRESSING

FOR STUDENTS.

BY

Mons. A. MALLEMONT

(PARIS),

President of La Société de Secours Mutuels des Coiffeurs de Paris
(Saint Louis et Union);

Member of L'Académie Ecole Française de Coiffure;

Conseiller Prud'homme du Département ae la Seine.

CONTAINING 56 ILLUSTRATIONS.

LONDON:

OSBORNE, GARRETT & Co., 51 & 52, FRITH STREET, SOHO, W.

1899.

PREFACE.

THE instant and remarkable appreciation which M. Mallemont's lessons in the Art of Hairdressing received when published serially in the columns of THE HAIRDRESSERS' WEEKLY JOURNAL is ample justification, if justification be needed, for the publication in volume form of a work which, from the moment it first saw the light in Paris, took its place in the front rank of text books for students. We think it may be stated, without fear of contradiction, that no other work exists which equals this manual in the wealth of its teaching to young hairdressers intent upon becoming masters of their profession. By the aid of the following pages, an earnest learner can perfect himself step by step from the primary and elementary stage of acquiring a knowledge of how to properly hold the comb to the building up of an elegant and artistic *coiffure.*

So much for the book itself, to which we may perhaps be permitted to add a few words of advice from the author to students entering, or who have already entered, the hairdressing profession. The proper inculcation of the principles laid down, is, perhaps, almost as indispensable to complete success, as the most profound knowledge of the technique of the art and natural skill. M. Mallemont says :—

"Young men who wish to enter the profession, must possess or acquire many qualities. It is not enough to become a good workman, although that is the first quality; but it is to his interest that the young man should have a good presence, be well dressed and extremely cleanly.

The hands should be well kept; the smell of tobacco should be entirely absent, as well as all other penetrating odours and perfumes.

Being called upon, when an artist in his work, to dress the heads of the highest ladies' in the land, he should possess sufficient tact not to let the want of education—if there be such—become apparent.

He should be very polite, and in conversation with his clients he should take great care not to offend against their religious or political opinions.

I must add, that perfect discretion as regards the secrets of his clients is quite indispensable."

It is unnecessary for us to add anything to these words of wisdom, but to cordially commend both them and the book to our many friends in the Hairdressing Trade.

THE PUBLISHERS.

CHAPTER I.

To Comb and Brush the Hair.

THE way to set about combing the hair, the ability shown in this initial operation, the manner in which the comb is held—all this is of great importance, and the customer, without seeming to pay attention to it, judges by such seemingly unimportant preliminaries as to the degree of confidence she may place in the professional knowledge of her hairdresser.

To comb the hair it is necessary, and it facilitates the work, for the client to be seated on a chair of ordinary height, and, if possible, before a glass with her face to the window. Having placed a cloth covering on the shoulders, the middle of the comb is held between the forefinger and the thumb of the right hand; the hair is thrown back; the left hand is placed at the back, underneath the hair, which is taken up by it and firmly held, and close to the head, so as to avoid the movements of the comb being felt. The combing should commence at the points and continue to the roots, in order that the operation may be done thoroughly and without pain; the left hand being especially occupied in dealing with any obstruction the comb may meet with.

The hairdresser should always place himself at a certain distance either behind or at the side, so as to be free in his movements without discomforting the customer. He should be quick, in order to avoid irritating the lady's nerves.

In brushing the hair, it should be separated into three or four divisions. Commencing from the roots, the brush should glide above and below the hair easily, so as to cause no inconvenience to the client.   Should the hair be dry, it is advisable to pour a few drops of brillantine into the

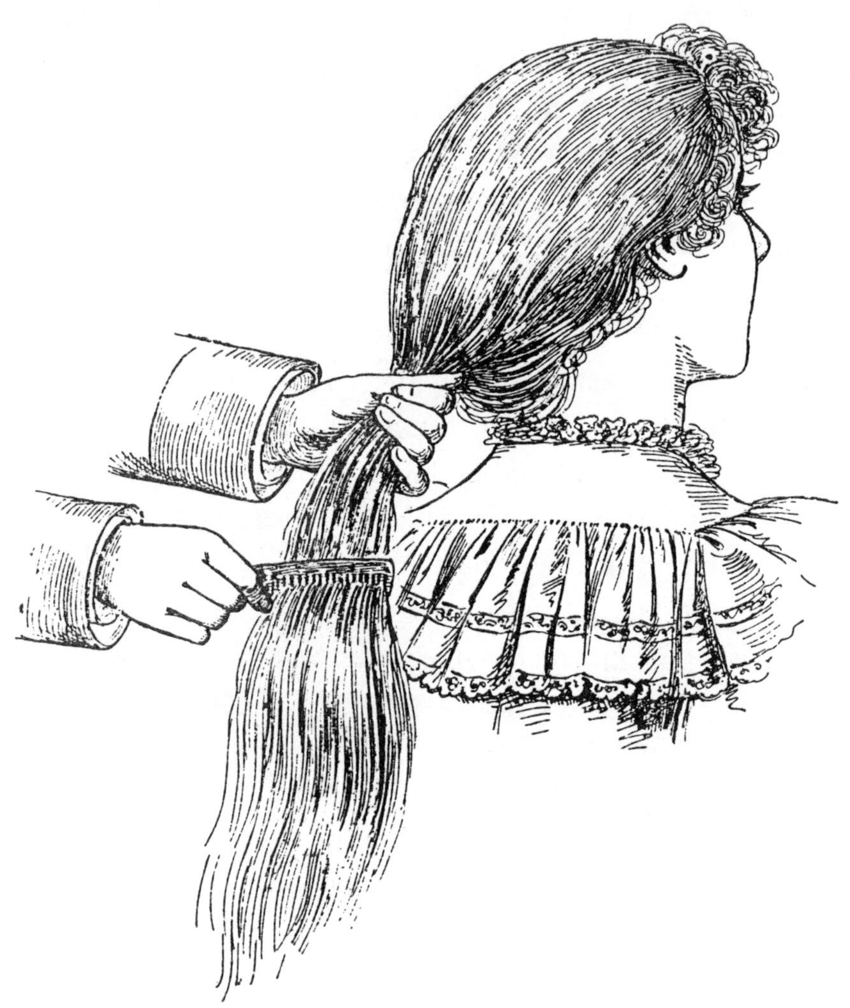

COMBING THE HAIR.

hollow of the hand (or else on to a brillantine brush), and apply it on top and underneath, until the hair acquires the necessary softness and sheen.

THE PARTINGS.

The first thing to learn is to trace a correct middle-parting, and then the cross-parting from ear to ear.   For

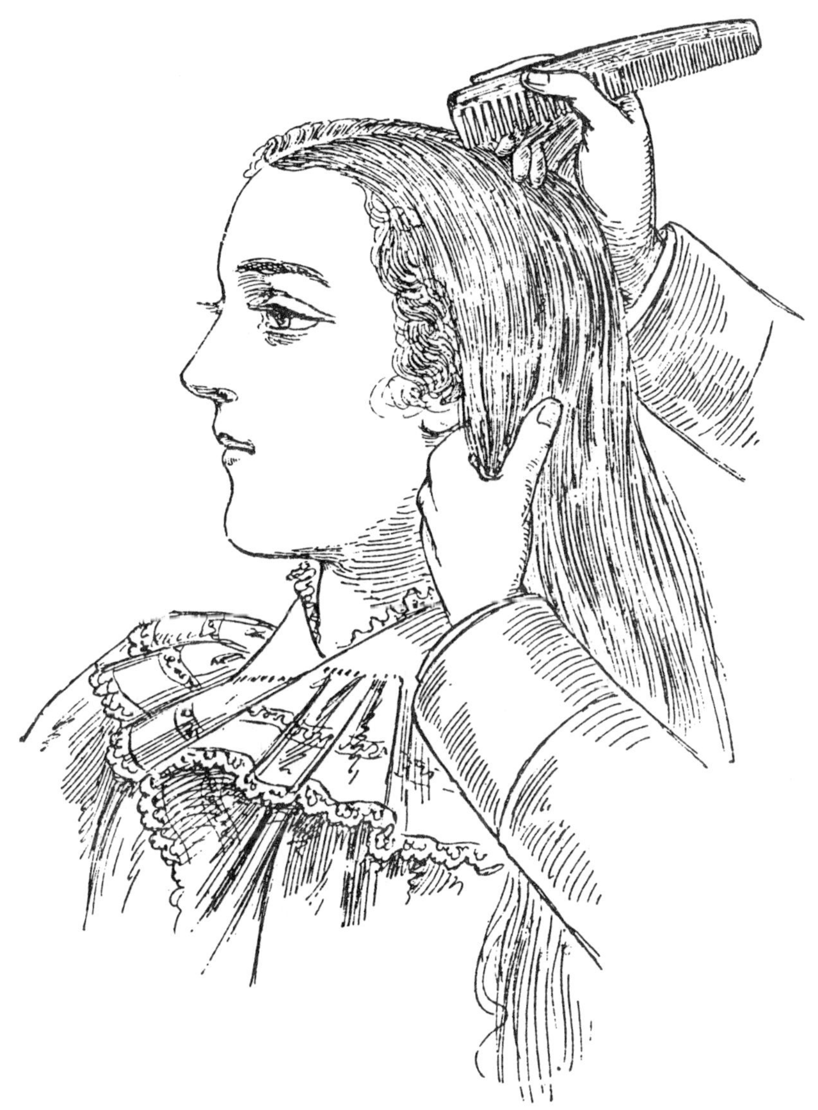

MAKING THE PARTING (CROSS-PARTING).

the middle-parting, the whole of the hair should be thrown back, and—the comb being held in the right hand—it should be combed back quite straight, the fine teeth of the comb pointing upwards. The parting should commence from the front with the first tooth of the comb, and should go right down to the neck. For the cross-parting, the hair should be combed down the sides, beginning at the middle parting in straight line behind the ear, the left hand holding the hair the while, and the thumb of that hand guiding the tooth of the comb.

The opposite side is parted in the same way. A hair-dresser who can do these two principal partings, will find no difficulty in doing other partings at the side or back of the head.

CUTTING THE HAIR.

It frequently happens that the hair splits at the points, or is of uneven length. In this case the cutting of the hair becomes necessary. It is done as follows :—

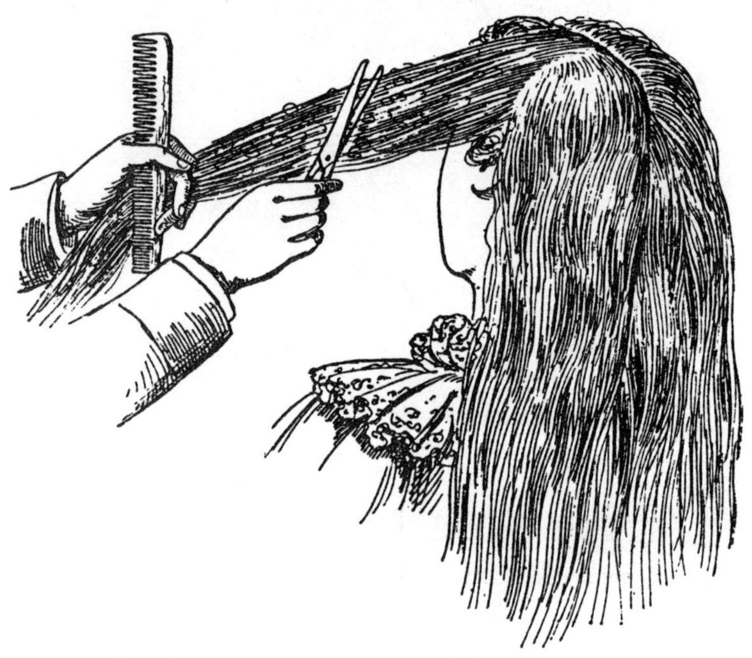

CUTTING THE HAIR.

Having combed out the hair, it is divided into several sections; each one in turn is held between the first two fingers of the left hand, and the points are brought out and cut in order to obtain the desired regularity of length. Having treated each piece in this way, the whole of the hair is combed and spread out on the shoulders, which will show whether any irregularity exists between the respective lengths of each section.

SINGEING THE HAIR.

When the hair splits at the ends, singeing is to be recommended. The ends are singed with a thin taper, or with apparatus specially made for the purpose.

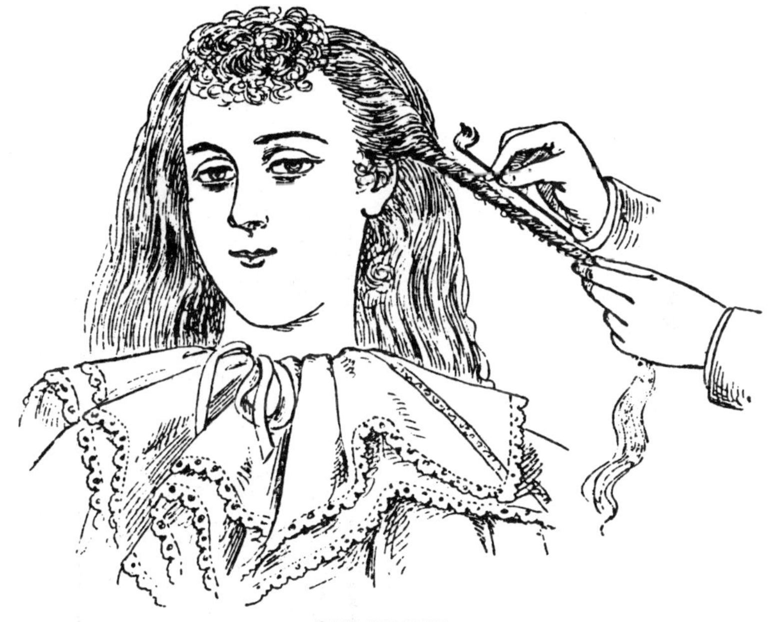

SINGEING.

The hair is divided as before, each piece being firmly held, the ragged points raised, and the flame passed along the points, so that all are singed. Care should be taken to hold the hair firmly, to prevent its catching fire.

Cleansing the Head by Friction.

For purposes of friction, specially prepared lotions are used ; they are applied with a sponge or with a bandoline brush with pointed handle. Commencing on one side of the head, the operation is continued right round to the other side, so that every part gets well cleansed.

Shampooing.

The hair should be carefully combed, and shampooed from root to point with the shampoo wash ; it should then be rinsed with tepid water, until the water running off is quite clear. If the client does not object, the operation should be finished with cold water. The hair can be dried partially with a Turkish towel, by twisting the towel round it and wringing. A hair-drying machine or some hot towels, will accomplish the remainder.

CHAPTER II.

Fastening the Hair.

TO properly execute a *coiffure*, as soon as the hair is combed and parted, a fastening has to be made. There are four principal ways of making a fastening: the bind, the plait, the 8, and the twist. The bind is made with a piece of ribbon about 16 inches long. Holding the hair in the left hand, with the thumb on the top (care should be taken that the hair is well combed and straight), one end of the ribbon is placed underneath the thumb, the ribbon being twisted round and round the hair, close up to the head, in spiral form. This prevents any pain being caused, while at the same time a firm fastening is obtained. The ends of the ribbon are then tied. If ribbon is not at hand, a piece of the hair may be used; it is wound round the hair in the same way as the ribbon, the ends being twisted round a hairpin stuck in at the end of the fastening.

In most of the present-day *coiffures* the fastening consists of a plait arranged just behind the crown. This plait serves to hold the hairpins by which the bandeaux are secured, and to fix more rigidly the ornamental comb, or pins, which hold up the hair combed from the neck.

Sometimes the fastening is made with a piece of hair of about the thickness of the little finger, which is twisted and shaped into a small 8. It is kept in shape by placing two hairpins crosswise, and twisting the hair round them, as well as the hair of the bandeaux, keeping the latter closely together, like the rest of the *coiffure*.

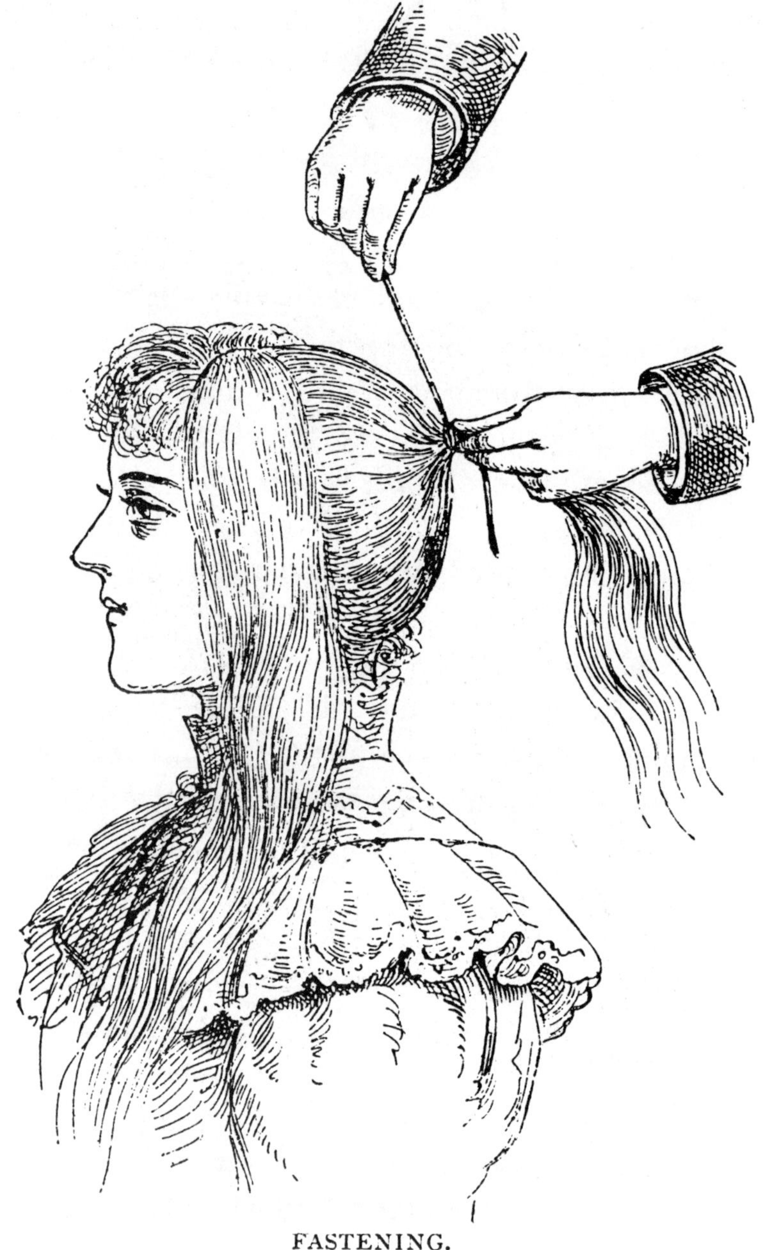

FASTENING.

By the twist the hair can be fastened without interfering

with the parting, and only a few inches in length are
sacrificed by its use. The hair is twisted for about three
or four inches, and lifted up straight, after being divided
into two portions, one being held by the left hand, while
the right hand makes half a turn, forming a ring, as seen in

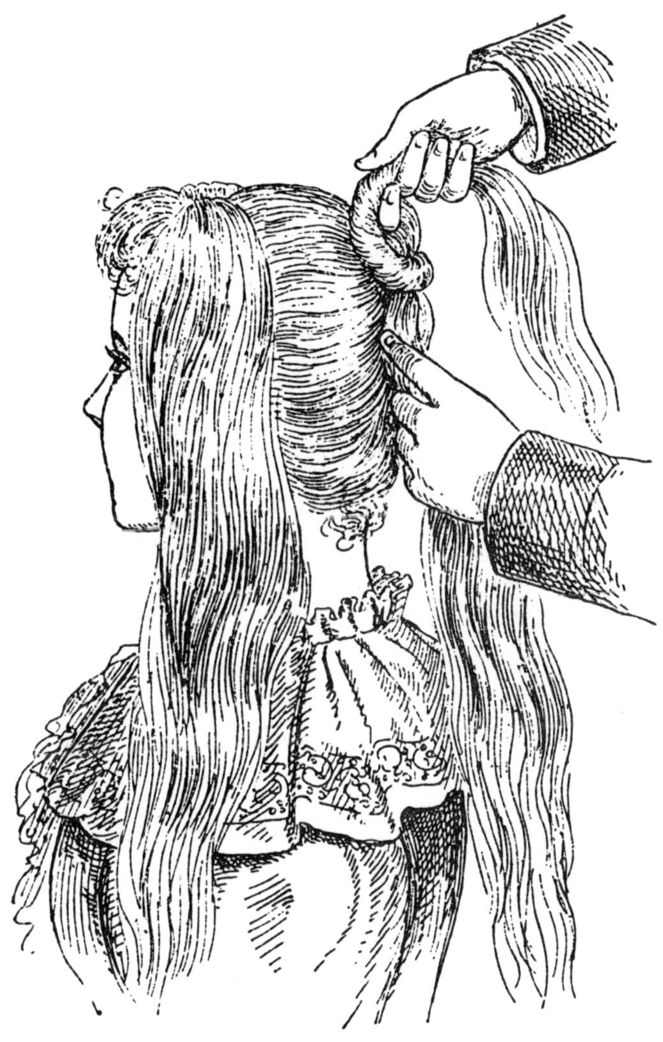

THE TWIST.

the design. A braid-comb, or two hairpins placed **X** shape,
hold the twist together.

CHAPTER III.

THE first part of the *coiffure* for the hairdresser to study and learn perfectly is the coil, for many of the operations performed in making it, recur in almost all other parts of the head-dress. As a *coiffure per se* it is only worn by a few elderly ladies; but, for the reason given above, it is indispensable that the hairdresser should know it thoroughly.

Since it frequently happens that the lady's own hair is insufficient, the operator should learn to add a piece of postiche, or a plait, and mingle it so carefully that it appears a part of the natural hair. To execute this operation well, the hair should be held in the palm of the left hand, between the thumb and three fingers, the forefinger pointing towards the head. The false piece should be held by the right hand, with the forefinger stretched out, the tip touching the loop of the false piece, and carefully introducing it between the natural hair. The left hand meanwhile should glide down, at the same time turning the hair, so as to cover regularly the additional piece, and enable the whole to be combed out together and made into a very even and smooth twist. Once the hair is twisted to the end, it is taken up straight, made into a snail-shaped coil, being finally fastened with a chignon comb, or with hair-pins.

In order to produce the 8, proceed in the same way as

with the coil, but when the twist is lifted up it is held at
the end with the left hand, while the right hand executes

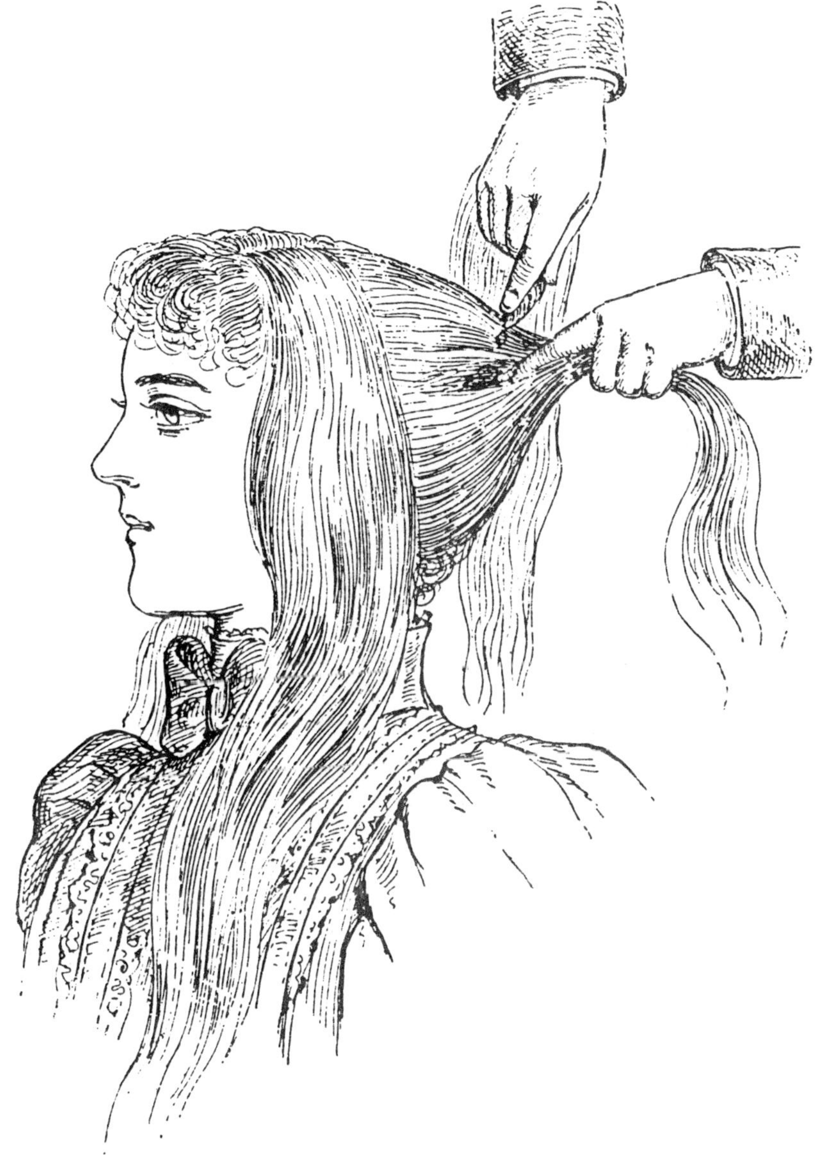

INTRODUCING A FALSE PIECE.

half a turn, forming a ring on the right; the left hand, at
the same time, forming a ring on the left. The 8 is made

as high up as required, and is fastened in the same way as the coil, with a chignon, or a braid comb, in the middle.

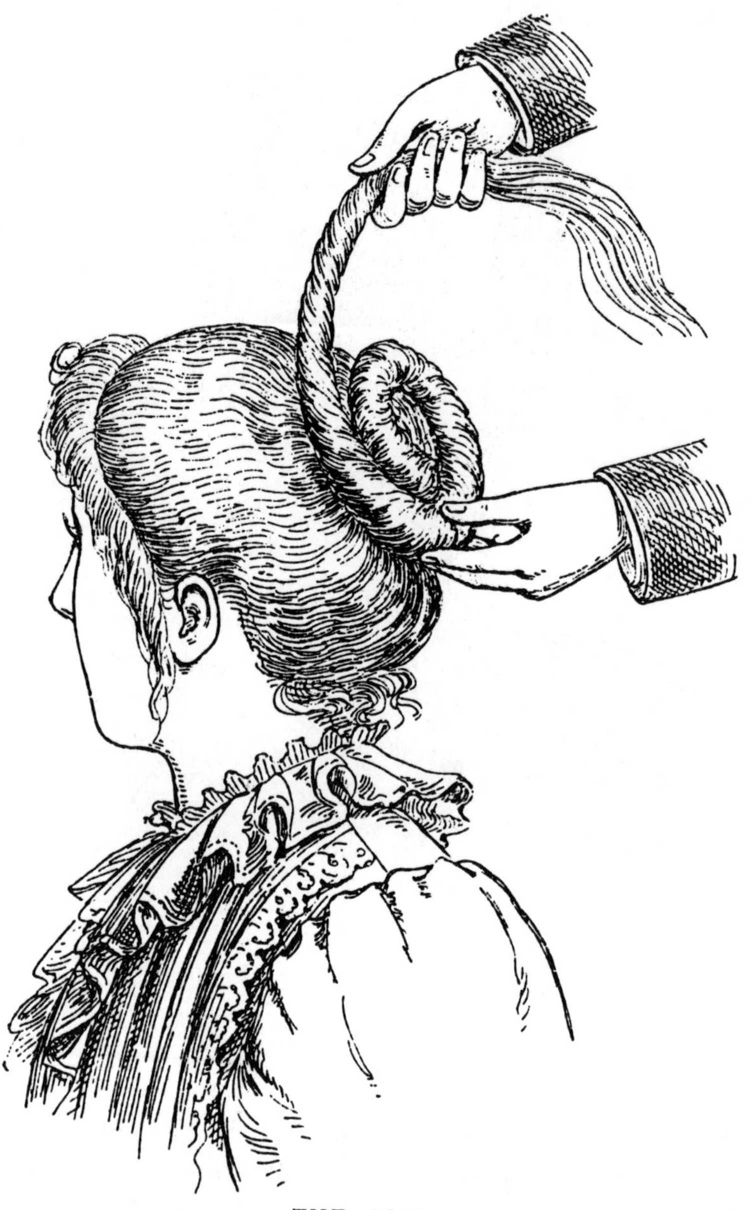

THE COIL.

To keep the 8 in good shape each loop of it should be pinned on well at the sides.

The twist is made with two pieces of hair of equal proportions, which are twisted towards the right, and, at the same time, round one another. To begin with, the right

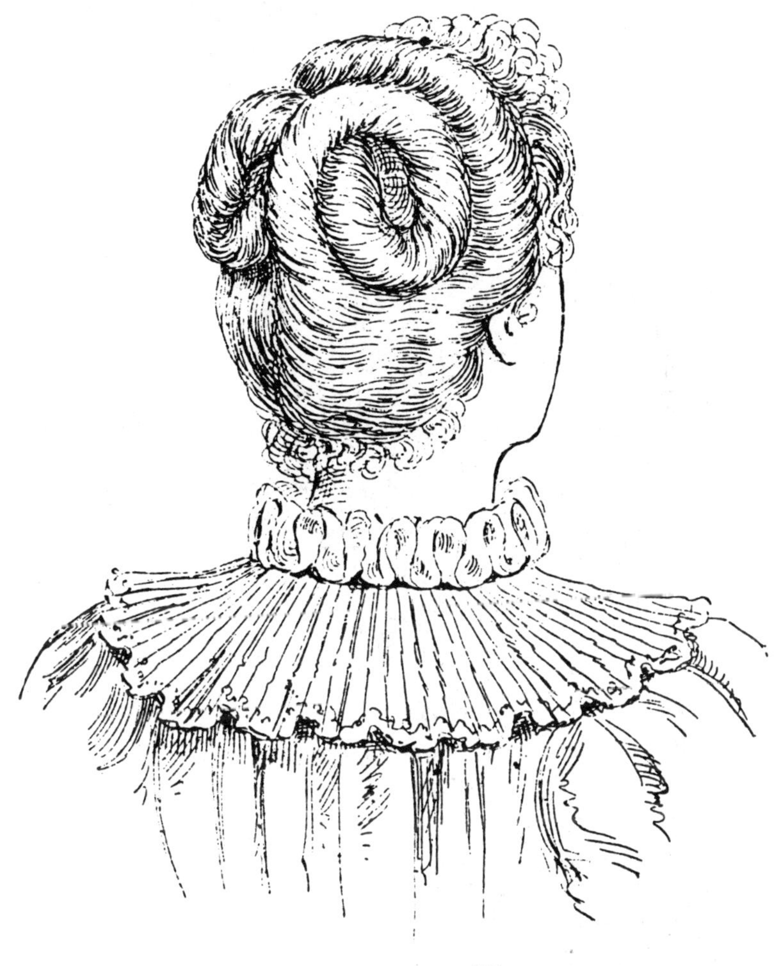

THE EIGHT (8).

twist. is passed over the left one. A twist may also be produced with a single piece by doubling it up, and then twisting it the same as the other. The plait is generally made of three pieces, which cross one another; they may be made with four, five, or even more pieces.

CHAPTER IV.

GORDIAN KNOT, GRECIAN KNOT, APOLLO KNOT.

THE *coiffures* most in favour with ladies are often the simplest; they are made by a turn of the hand and elegantly manipulated. We shall describe several kinds of arrangements—in fact, those mostly employed.

The Gordian knot is, above all, used when the hair-dresser wishes to reduce the volume of a too abundant head of hair, as well as its extreme length. With this knot the chignon can be made and the sides garnished; it can further easily be shaped in diadem form.

The Gordian knot is made with a rather thick piece of hair, which being held by the right hand at the end, should be twisted; then, with the left hand, the palm of which is placed underneath, half a turn is made to produce a loop. The right hand then passes the end of the piece through the loop, and the piece is allowed to drop down as indicated in the design.

The Grecian knot, fashionable for several years, serves to form the chignon and is very easy of execution. Having twisted the hair, it is sufficient to form half an eight on the right, and to pass the twist on the neck through the middle, taking care to give it a good shape. Should the

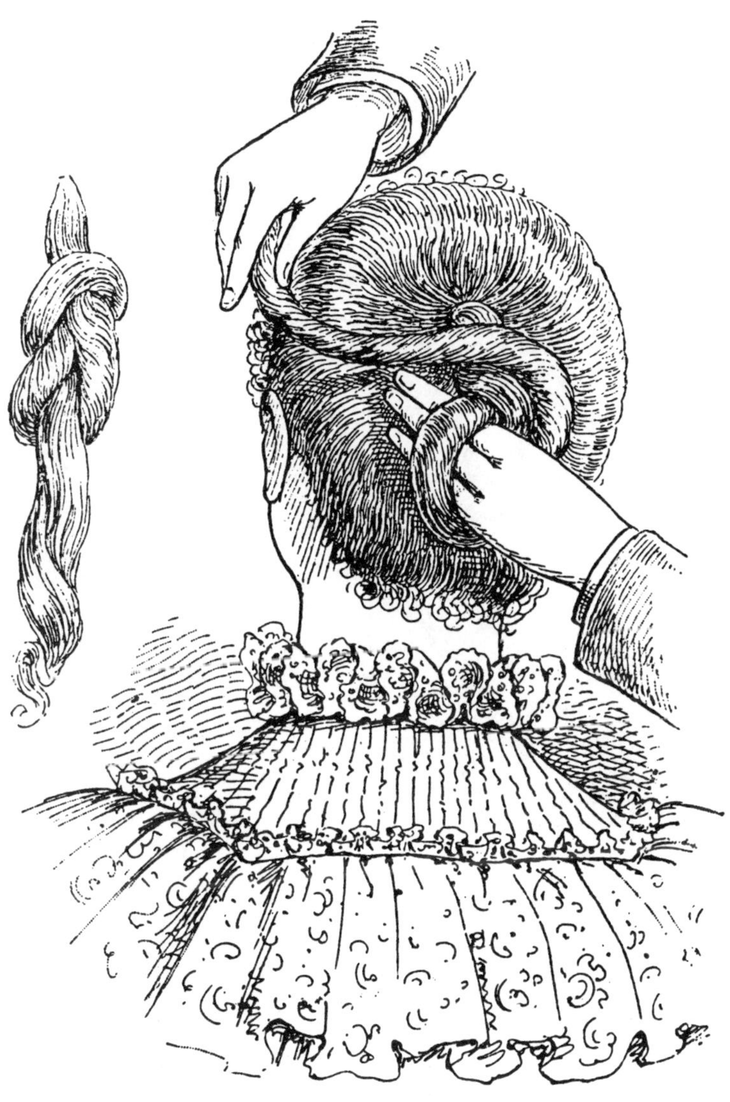

THE GORDIAN KNOT.

hair be very long, it should be twisted and rolled round this knot in regular layers.

The Apollo knot is a large bow *(coque girafe)* tied at the bottom ; it can be placed on the crown, or lower down, to form the chignon, like the Grecian knot.   The way to

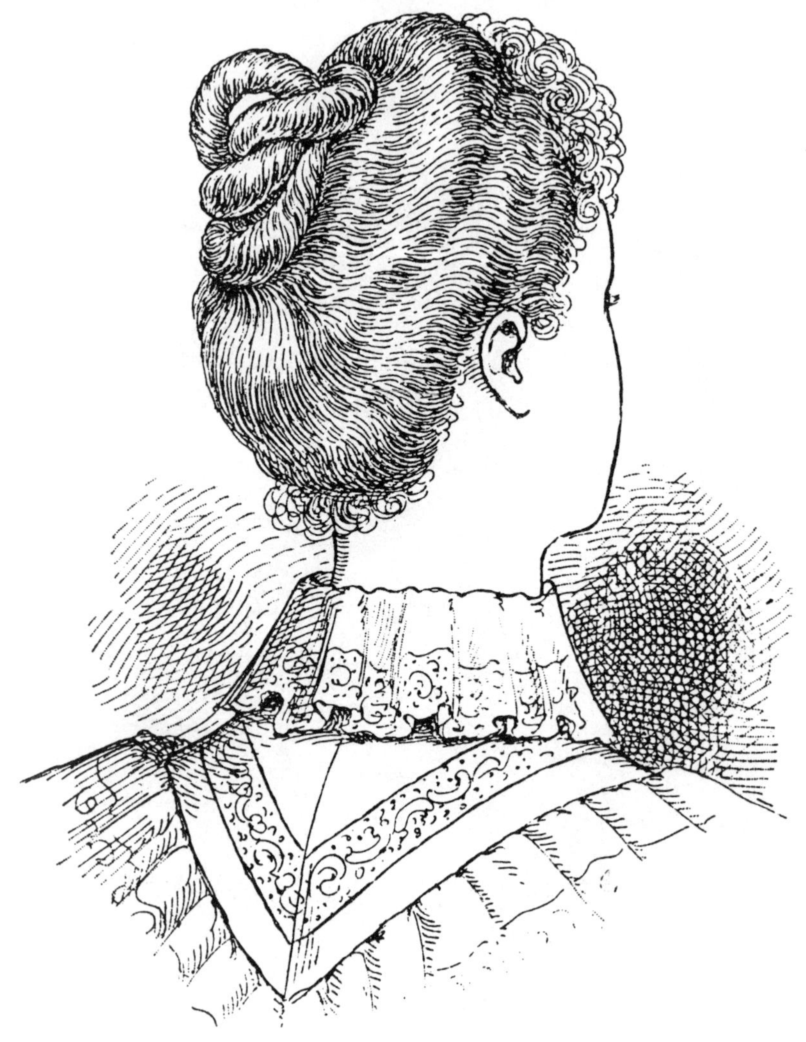

THE GRECIAN KNOT.

make the Apollo knot is as follows : Arrange the hair flat like a ribbon, hold the points with the left hand, place the first three fingers of the right hand underneath in the middle, give half a turn and form a loop; then pass the

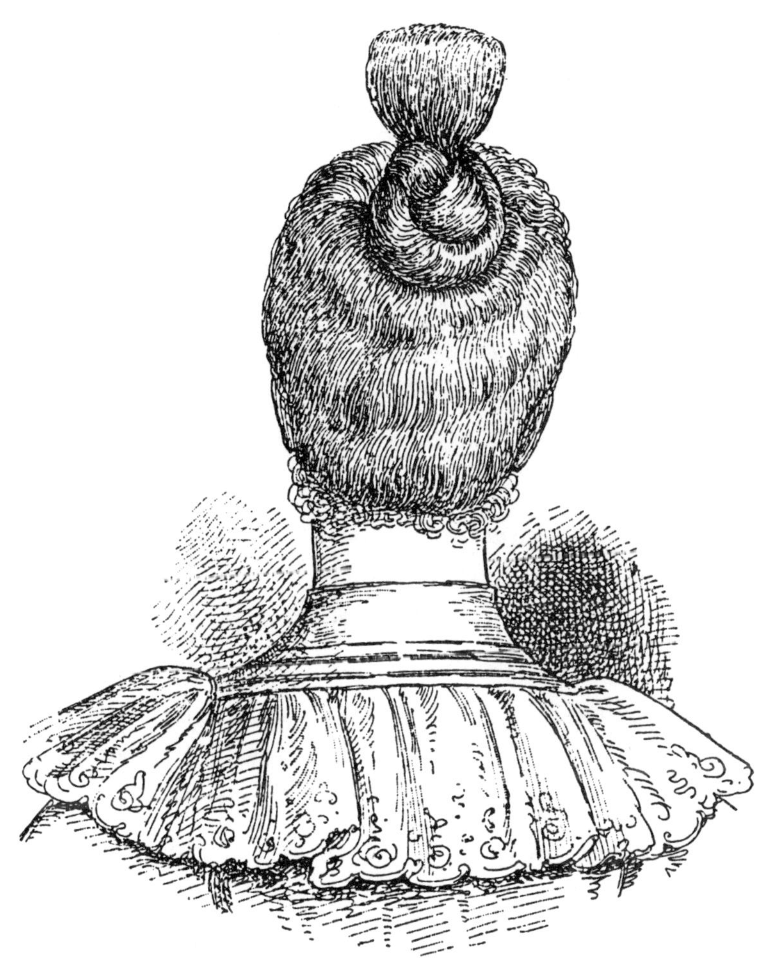

APOLLO KNOT.

lower end through the loop, taking care that it forms a flat loop; tighten by drawing the ends with the left.

CHAPTER V.

IT is necessary to crimp the hair underneath for bows, when the latter are to be puffy, and especially when the hair is thin. It is therefore important to know how to crimp well. Take the hair between the first and second fingers of the left hand flattened like a ribbon, and hold it straight. The comb is held in the right hand, and only the fine teeth are used for crimping; in short, regular strokes from root to point, the hair should be combed; if not sufficiently crimped, commence again regularly from top to bottom. The hair can easily be uncrimped by using the coarse part of the comb, and combing in the reverse direction—viz., from point to root.

If you wish to make marteaux bows, divide the hair into as many pieces as the number of bows required. Each piece of hair should be combed flat, and slightly crimped. Take one piece between the thumb and second finger of each hand, glide down to the points, and roll up more or less tightly, according to the size of the bow required.

With the bow made with the raised hand, *coiffures* of the 1830 style can be arranged. With the *girafe* bow very light *coiffures* may be obtained; the many bows giving an elegant shape, and the impression of a curled head-dress. This bow is made as follows: Having divided the hair into the necessary pieces, each piece is taken up with the left hand, three fingers of the right hand are placed underneath, half a turn is given, and the hair is fastened tightly at the root of the bow. It is possible, also, to make several bows with the piece, if the hair is long enough, by pinning the hair up at equal distances into loops, giving each time half a turn with a pin to form the loop.

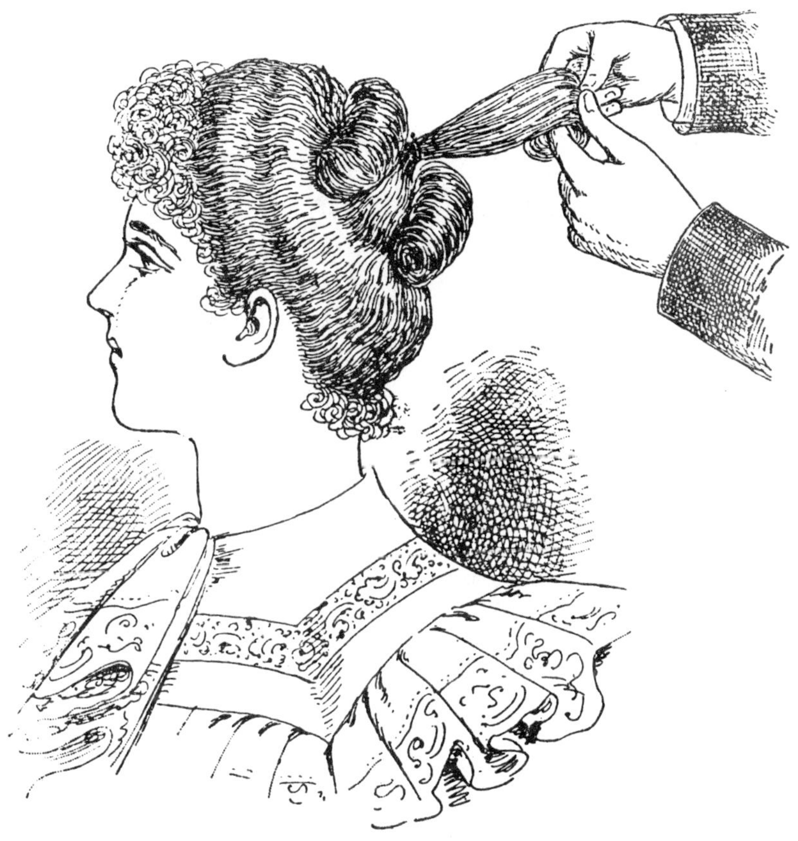

MARTEAU BOW.

There are many other ways to arrange bows, but they are not often employed. There is, for instance, the Marie Antoinette bow, which is made by rolling the hair round all the fingers of the left hand. The hair should be well frizzed.   According to the length of the hair, a single piece

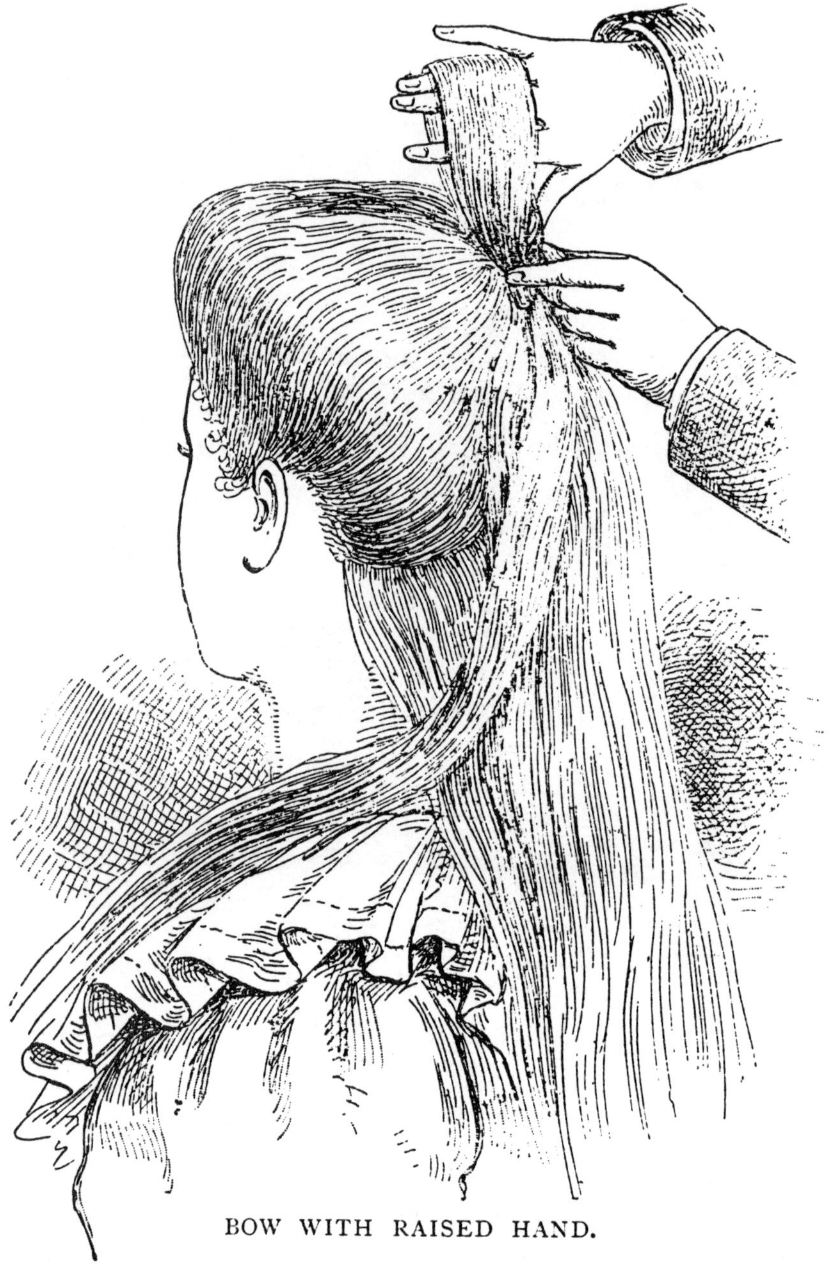

BOW WITH RAISED HAND.

is often sufficient for several pinned bows, by making for
each bow a half turn with the hairpin.

CHAPTER VI

RAISED BANDEAUX, RAISED POMPADOUR, RAISED
BANDEAUX, STYLE LOUIS XV.

WHEN the front hair is combed back, either parted in the middle (Marie Stuart style) or without parting (Pompadour or Marie Antoinette style), it is necessary to crimp the hair to make it bulge, and very often a suitable frizzett is placed underneath the hair. The frizzetts should be made with great care, especially where the client's hair is thin. By preference, these frizzetts should be mounted on combs—the hair, if possible, being knotted. In placing the frizzetts, you lift the natural hair with the left hand, holding it well up, and rather forward; and with the right hand you push in the comb of the frizzett at the foot of the raised hair, as shown in the design. The hair is then spread over it with the palm of the left hand, and combed with the fine side of the comb.

To make raised bandeaux (Marie Stuart style), begin by getting the front and cross-partings, then make a fastening, crimp the hair, or else place the frizzett. Taking the hair in the palm of the hand, glide the forefinger of the right hand underneath, pressing the hair the while with the thumb. Still gliding, give half a turn and fasten the bandeau with a hairpin, being careful to take the hair to the fastening point.

The Pompadour bandeau : Make a slanting front-parting ;

commence by combing up the hair at both sides, straight over the frizzetts; and after it has been secured at the

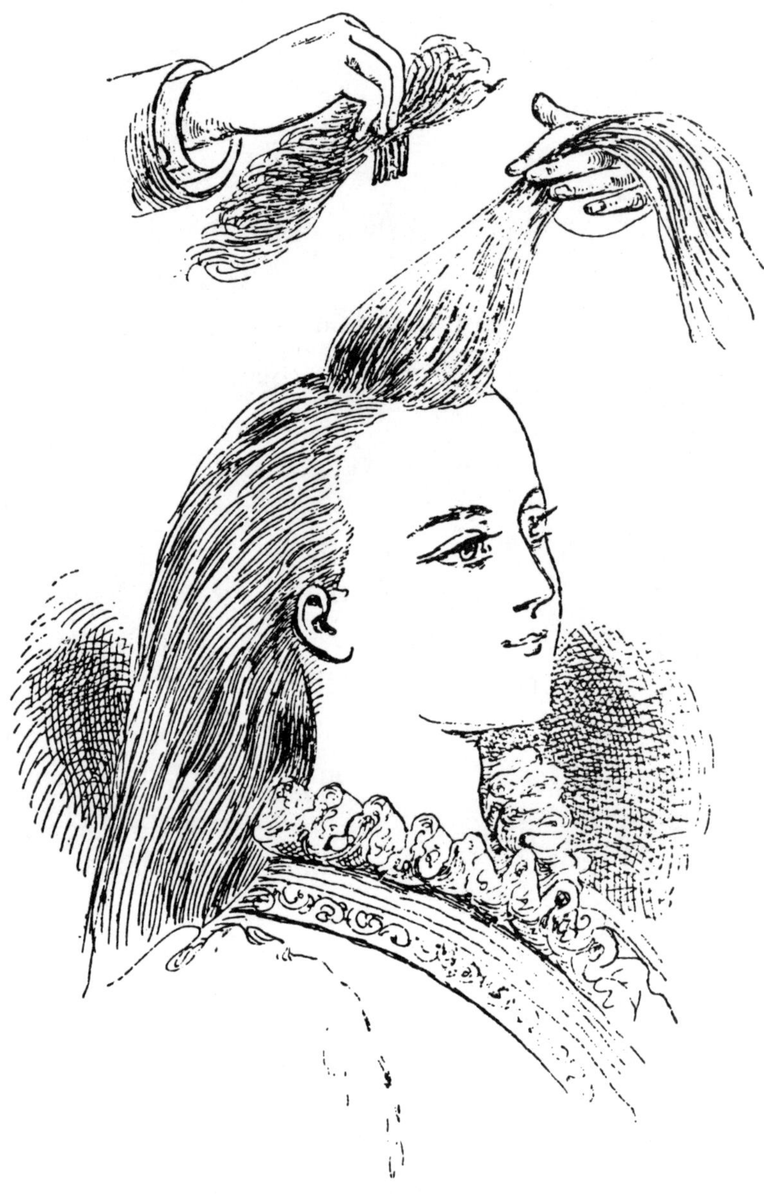

PLACING A FRIZZETT ON COMB.

fastening point, comb up the front hair quite straight, and the slanting parting will prevent any separation of the hair.

The Marie Antoinette is made in the same manner, only the frizzetts are much larger.

The Louis XV. bandeaux, which are shaped like marteaux bows, require as many cross-partings from ear to

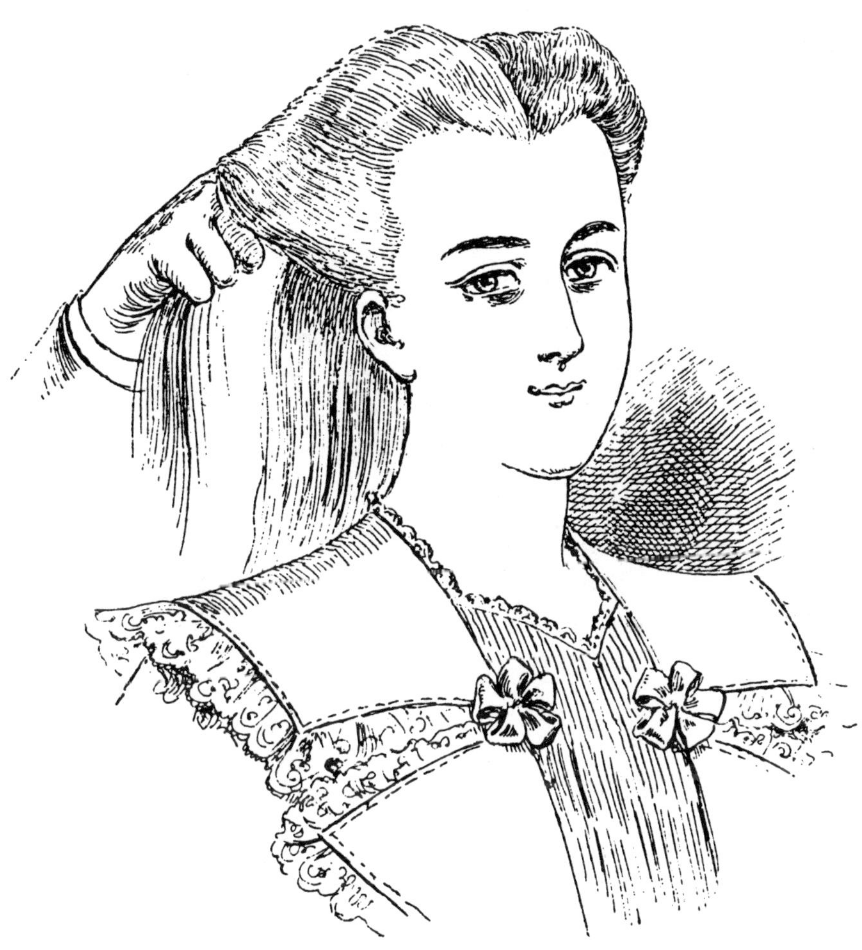

RAISED BANDEAU (MARIE STUART).

ear as bows are required (seven at least). The first bandeau is made on the middle of the forehead. Having slightly crimped the piece, take hold of it with the thumb and forefinger of the right hand, give half a turn upwards, gliding the finger so as to shape a rolled bandeau, which is pinned backwards to the fastening. The other bandeaux on either side are done in the same way. It is important, in executing this *coiffure*, to arrange the bandeaux so as to give a good shape to the head.

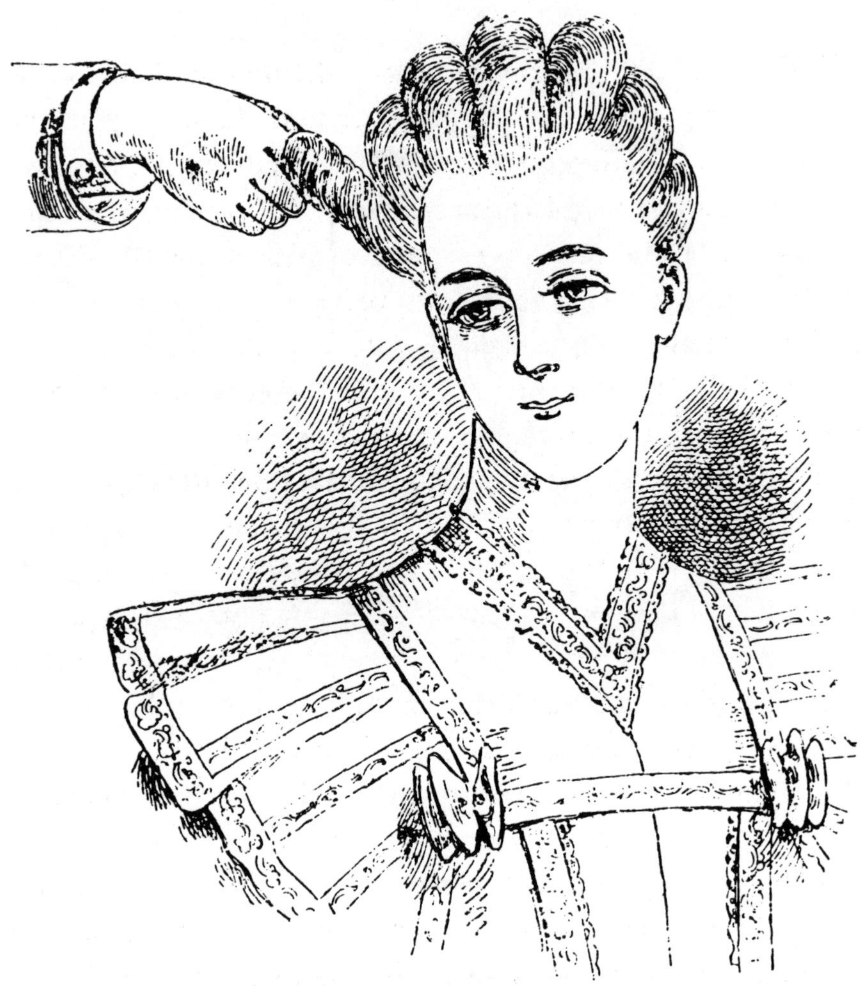

RAISED BANDEAU (LOUIS XV.)

CHAPTER VII.

VIRGIN MARY, EMPRESS, AND CLEO BANDEAUX.

TO make the Virgin bandeau, divide the hair, by a front parting, in two equal portions; make a plait on each side, well smoothing down the hair from the temples to the ears. The plaits may either fall down over the shoulders, or be pinned up at the neck, chignon shape. Another way is to make a front-parting, and cross-parting, and a fastening. It is sufficient to smooth the front hair down; bring up the ends as high as the ears and pin on to the fastening, and arrange a chignon.

THE EMPRESS BANDEAUX.—These bandeaux, which the Empress Eugenie wore, are executed differently. Having made a front and cross parting, reserve on each side of the former a fairly thick piece of hair, and separate it from the rest by a parting beginning from the cross parting and extending to the temple, the remainder of the hair being combed back and fastened together. To make this style of *coiffure*, frizzetts should be used as much as possible, particularly those knotted on slanting combs. Having placed them aside of the middle parting, take the hair between the thumb and the outstretched forefinger; do half a turn upwards over the index; while with the other hand give it the form of a ram's horn. The bandeau is then pinned behind the ear, and the ends are twisted round the fastening, which should be near the nape of the neck. Instead of frizzetts, large plaits mounted on combs may be used. They are placed in the same way, the ends being utilized to garnish the part behind the ears, as in the Italian *coiffures*.

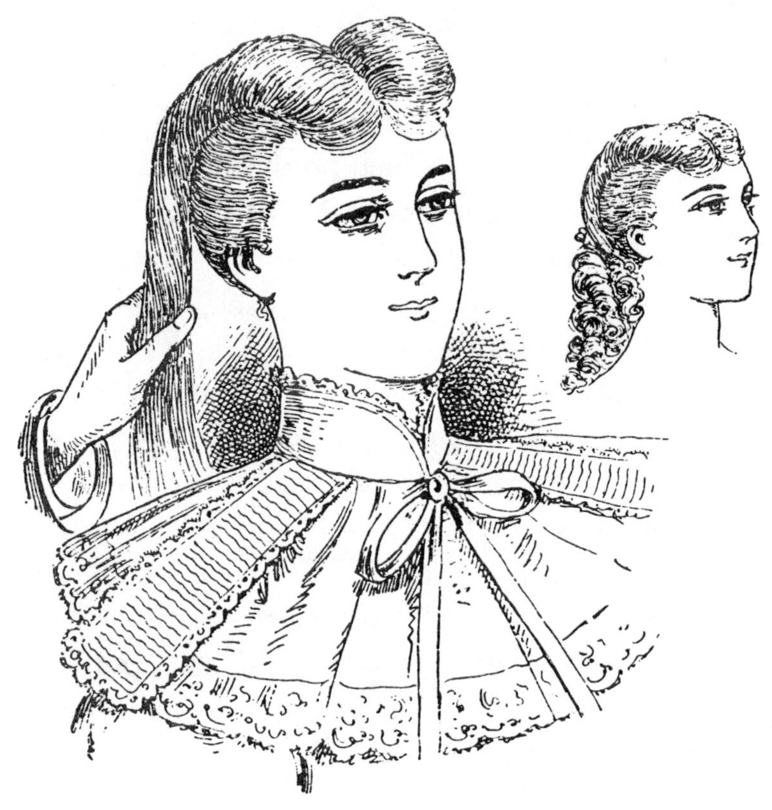

EMPRESS BANDEAU.

THE CLEO BANDEAUX.—Where the hair is not abundant it should be strongly crimped, unless under-bandeaux, or frizzetts, are preferred to cause the nair to bulge out. Make a middle parting; take hold of the whole of the hair with the left hand; smooth the hair down on each side of the forehead, covering the temples and ears completely. The two ends should then be loosely twisted, and the chignon formed at the nape of the neck.

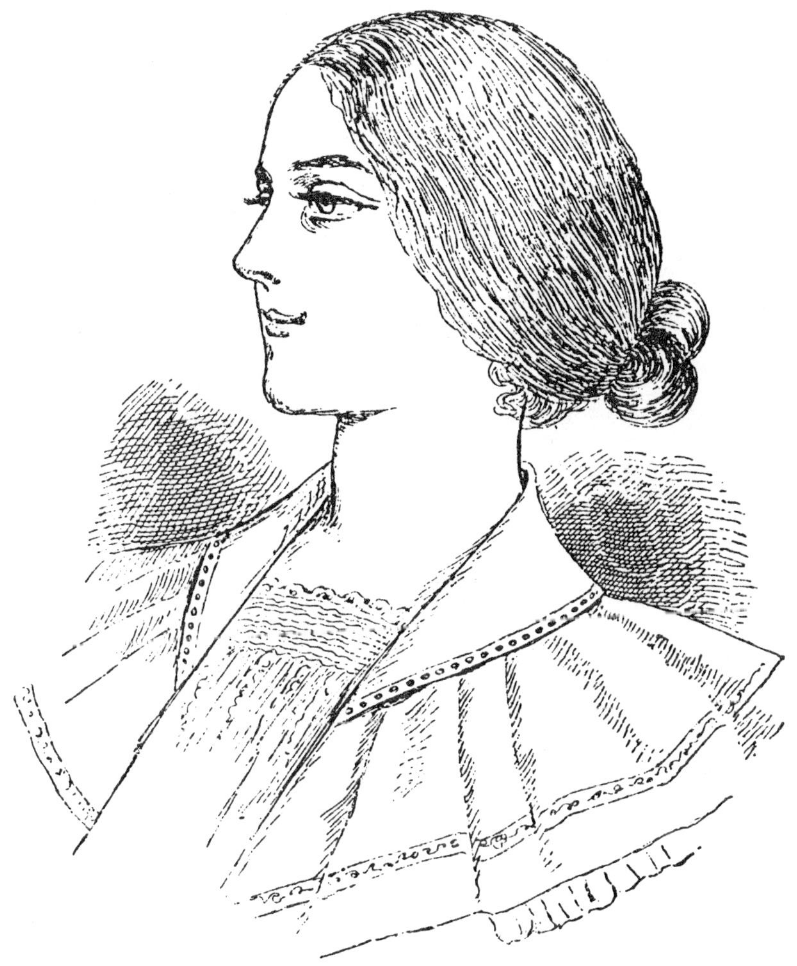

CLEO BANDEAU.

CHAPTER VIII.

SINCE the earliest ages, Grecian, as well as Roman, poets, painters, and sculptors, have testified to the charm imparted to female loveliness by curled hair. The legend of Queen Berenice tells us that that royal lady had a magnificent head of curls, which she sacrificed on the altar of Venus, in order to ensure the safety of her husband, Pholemacus Evergetes, against the perils of an expedition he was conducting in Syria. Callimachus, the poet laureate of the King's Court, continues the legend, in complicity with Samis, the astronomer, affirmed that the curls of the faithful Queen had had the supreme honour of being carried aloft to the heavens and changed into the constellation of stars, which to this day retains the name of the " Hair of Berenice."

Coiffures executed with curled hair constitute not only the latest fashion, but they have the advantage of being light, and generally speaking, more becoming than those made with straight hair. It is therefore indispensable that the hairdresser should know how to give straight hair the appearance of curled hair by curling, crimping, or waving it, and make it look exactly like the hair of persons who have natural curls.

PAPILLOTES OR RINGLET CURLS.—These are made as follows: Comb out the hair carefully, and make partings at regular intervals. Divide the hair into small pieces, according to the size of the curls and the thickness of the head of hair. The curling paper should be very soft

and cut into triangular shapes.   Commencing with the
piece near the middle parting, catch hold of the hair with
the thumb and forefinger and glide down to the points,
which make into round, tight rings, by using simultaneously
the right and left hands.   Continue rolling up towards the

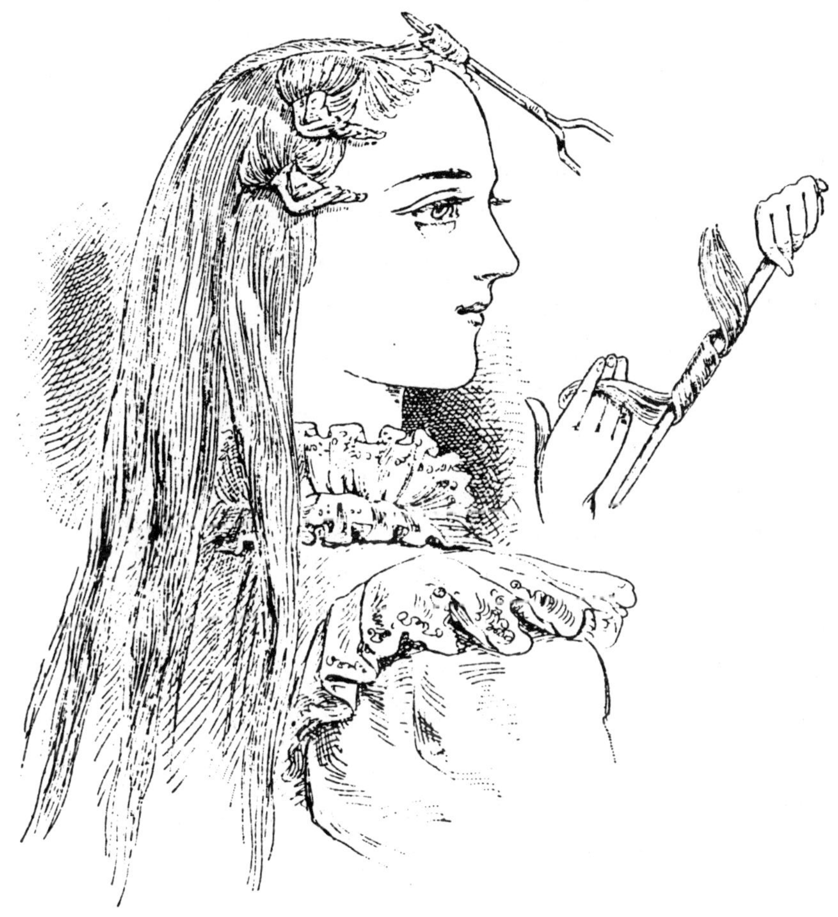

RINGLET CURLS.

roots so that you get a tightly made and almost flat ring.
That is the ringlet curl, which is then enveloped in the
paper; the paper is placed underneath the ring with the
right hand, the other hand holding the ringlet tightly.

The left corner of the paper is turned over first and held beneath the thumb, the right corner is next folded over the ring, until the whole is twisted round, when it is pressed with the pinching-iron.

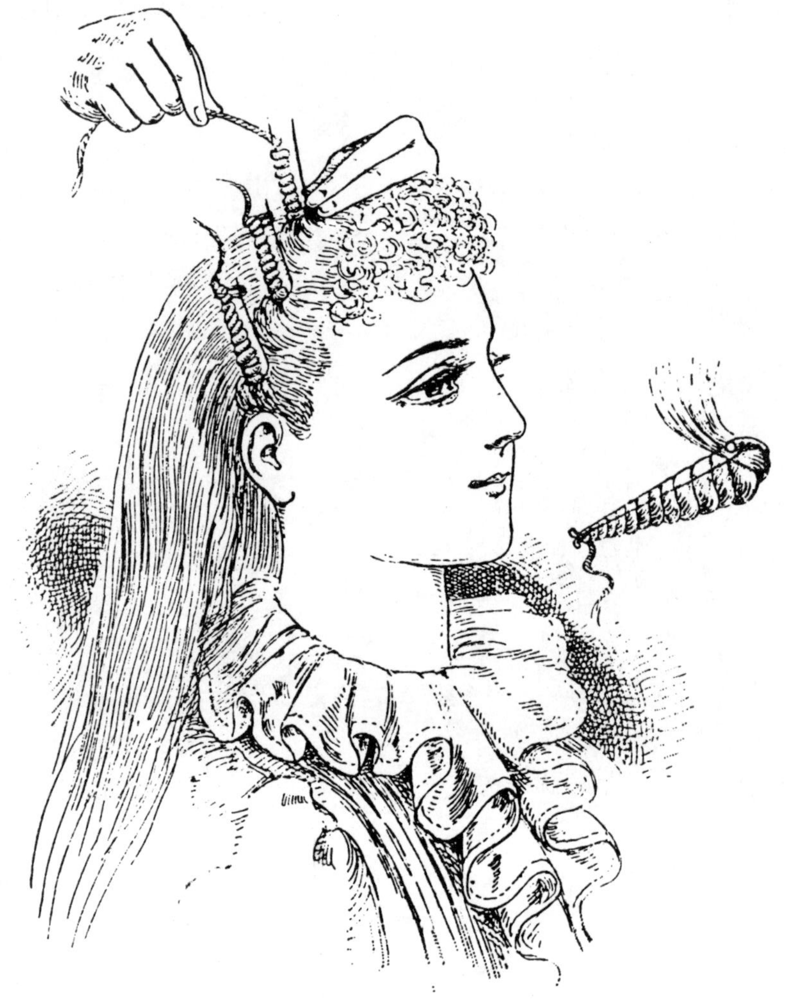

SPIRAL WAVING.

CURLED HAIR.—Curls can be made with leather rollers, or the curling iron; but it is better to put hair into curling-paper first and then use the iron. Where leather-rollers are used, the hair should be rolled over them from the extreme point to the roots. Short hair is best treated with the round iron. The hair is divided into small pieces; the thumb and forefinger of the left hand hold a piece, which is then put in the iron, the hollow prong upwards. Glide the iron down to the points, and roll the piece up tightly in the direction the curl is to be, leaving the iron in it for a few seconds. Open and shut the iron several times in turning it, seeing that the curl is perfectly round and that you can easily withdraw the iron. Care should be taken to see that the iron is properly heated, by trying it on a piece of white paper, which it should in no way discolour, or the hair will be burnt.

CURLS.—When the hair has cooled, it should be slightly frizzed, given the shape of a ribbon, and, held between the first two fingers, rolled over a curling-stick.

WAVES.—Make a parting right round the head about an inch from the forehead, according to the thickness of the hair to be waved. Divide the hair into small pieces (about ten) all round the head; twist each one and roll up tightly round one of the prongs of a hairpin spirally. Turn over the point of the pin, to hold the hair, then pinch with the iron. In order to get larger waves, thicker pieces of hair should be used. There are several kinds of pins to make these waves with.

WAVING ON HAIRPINS.—Flat waves on hairpins are more difficult to make and require great attention, if you wish to obtain an elegant *coiffure* with regular waves; and more difficult still when waved bandeaux are to be made, with light flat waves over the forehead. Pass the piece of hair to be waved between the prongs of the hairpin, holding it

between the thumb and forefinger, and winding it over the
two prongs in order to form 88, gently pushing the pin the
while.   Always keep the nail of the thumb in view, so that

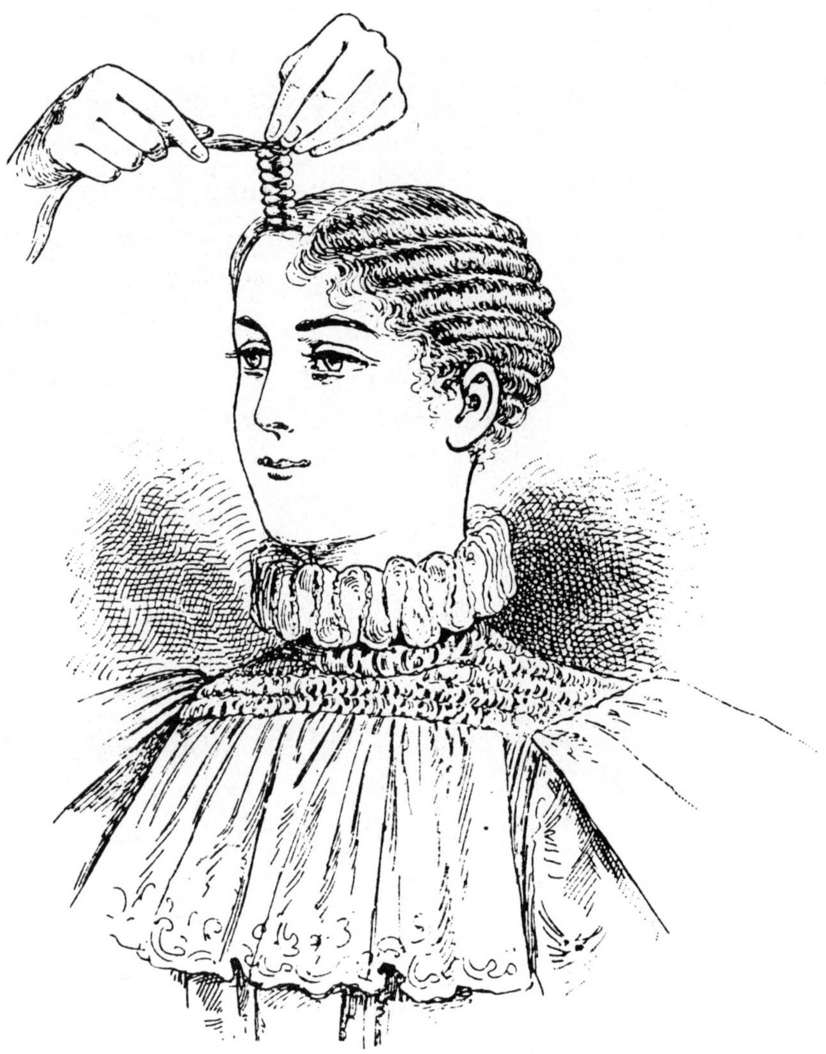

FLAT WAVING ON PIN.

the wave is quite flat and on the same side.   Then pinch
the hair with the iron.   To put the waved hair in place, it
should be combed slantingly and backwards, with a single

stroke of the comb if possible; and it will shape itself in very light waves over the forehead.

WAVING ON IVORY STICKS.—This mode of waving produces beautiful undulations, and may be resorted to when

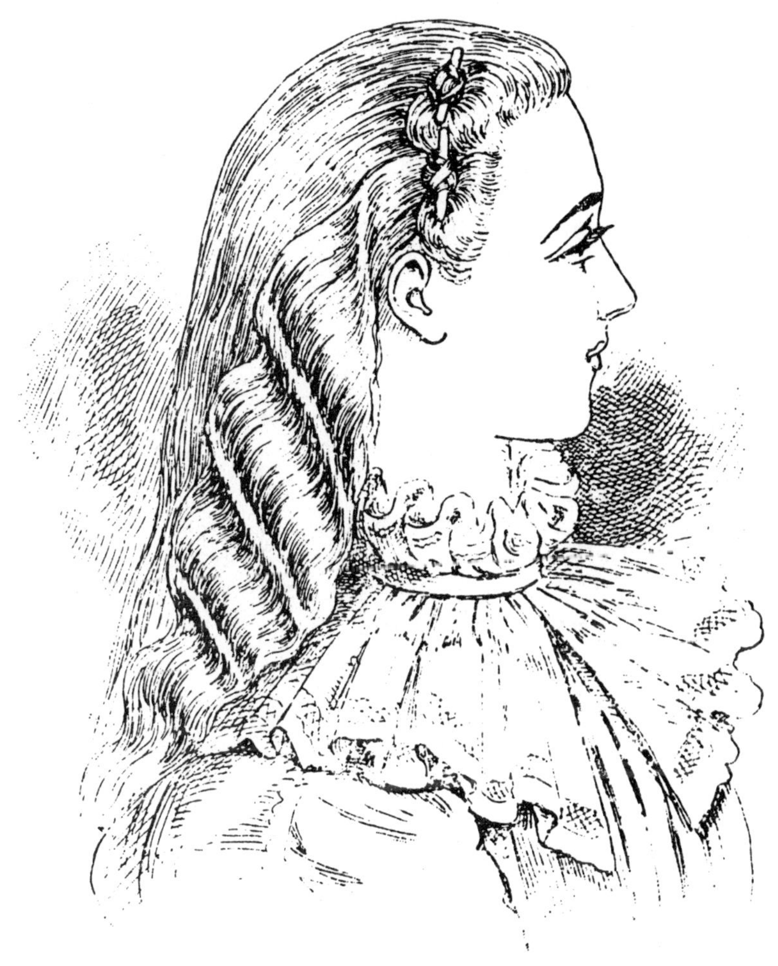

WAVING ON IVORY STICKS.

making the cross-bandeaux, which obtained such successful patronage at the end of the Empire. The sticks used are small, from two to two and a half inches long, and are flat, oval-shaped. The stick is placed across the roots underneath the hair; the piece, well flattened, is taken in the right hand and wound over the stick, crossing from right to left; the ends are secured by pinning them across; then pinch with the iron. One of the difficulties of this mode of waving is to get the waves to join one another properly; for that purpose it is necessary to make them all of exactly the same size, and to take in account the distances, which must be very even.

CHAPTER IX.

WAVING WITH THE IRON (MARCEL PATTERN); WAVED COIFFURE.

THE great success obtained by this style of waving is due to the fact that it gives straight hair the exact appearance of naturally waved hair; so much so, that ladies, whose hair is rather thin, appear, with this style of waving, to possess magnificent heads of waved hair— thanks to the art of the hairdresser. When well executed, the waves will last a fortnight; which is a great saving for clients, as the mere dressing of the hair takes much less time.

WAVING WITH THE IRON: For the purpose of getting the hair well waved, it should be clean and dry. We should advise the learner to begin on a piece of false hair. Let him divide it into three not very thick pieces; then take the uppermost piece, flattened ribbon shape, between the first and second fingers of the left hand. By a first upward move of the iron, waves are formed, the hair being kept close to the iron; by a second move, the iron glides down in the reverse direction, the left hand following the iron closely. The upward and downward moves produce the undulations; they are continued to the end of the piece, each set of motions forming a wave. When the learner has acquired the proper moves, he should try his hand on other pieces, always taking care that the waves of

all the pieces produce a continuous undulation. Only
after earnest study and repeated trials of the moves
indicated, should the operator proceed to execute this
undulation on the head of hair of a client.

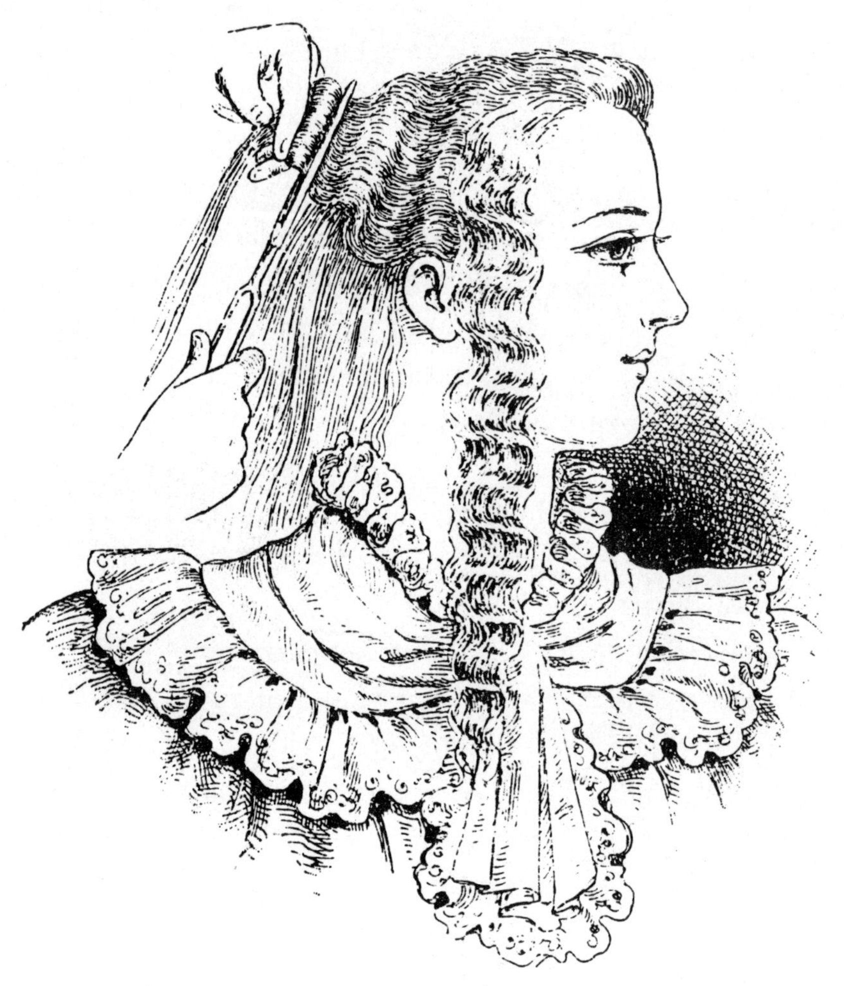

WAVING WITH THE IRON (MARCEL PATTERN).

In waving a lady's hair, you should invariably begin at
the right side, and the first wave should frame the ear,
leaving the roots to be waved last (see sketch above).
The alternate moves produce waves more or less large.

The first piece being waved through its entire length, a
small portion of it should be added to the next piece, to
serve as a guide for the waves in that, so that when the

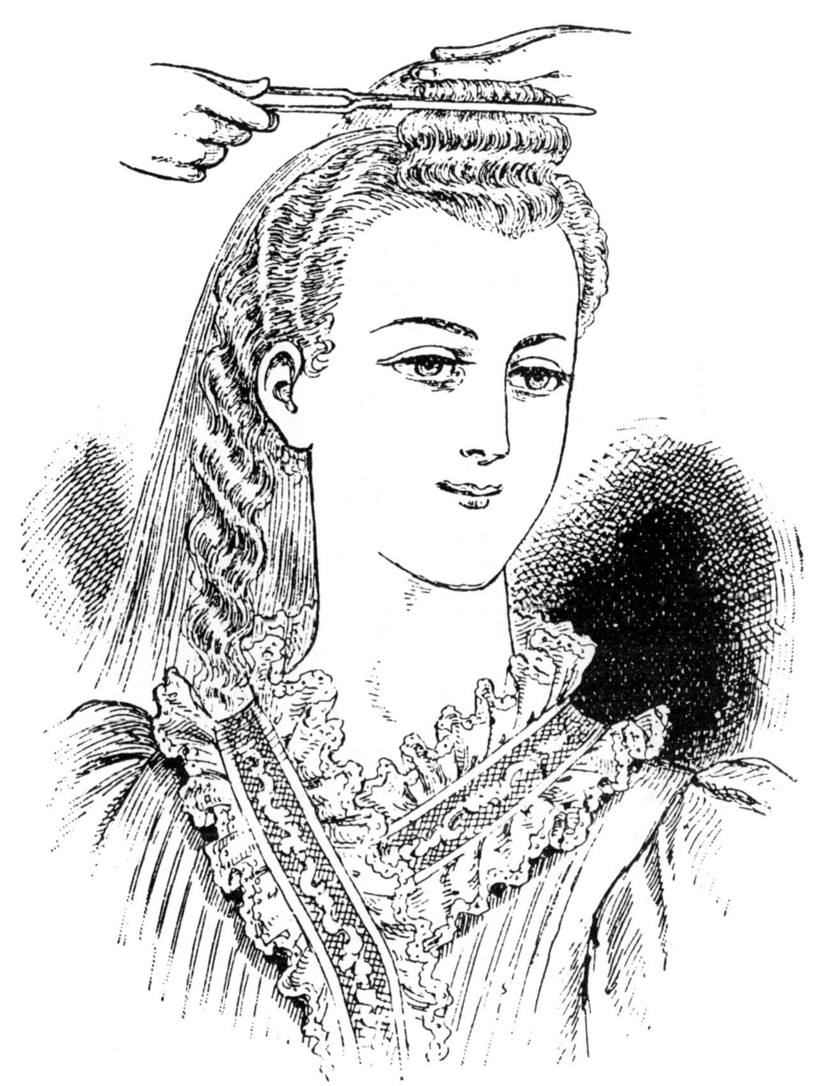

WAVING WITH THE IRON (MARCEL PATTERN).

whole of the hair is afterwards combed, the waves produce
an unbroken undulation right round the head. When the
right side is finished, the left should be taken in hand.

Let it be understood that the hollow part of the iron
should always be below. When both sides are finished,
the hair on the top of the head should be waved, and for
a guide here as to uniformity, a piece from the right side

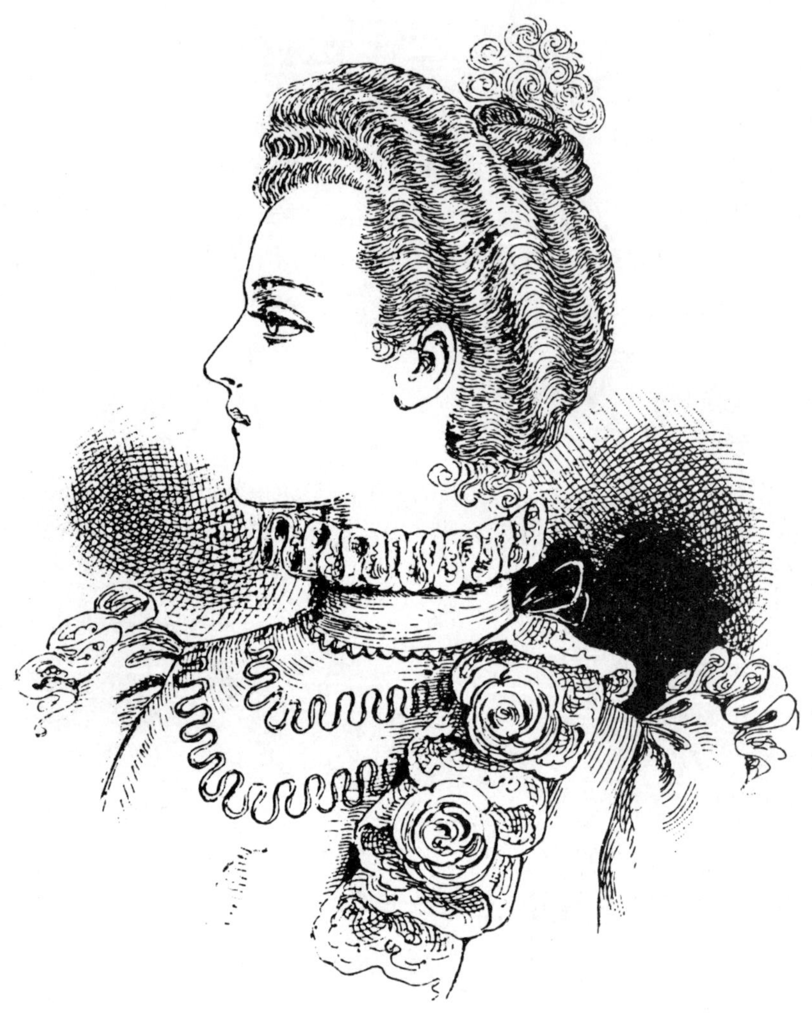

WAVED COIFFURE.

can be used. To wave the hair on the neck, the head
should be slightly bent forward. The whole of the hair,
being now waved, should be pinned at the top of the head.

Take the pieces in their turn between the thumb and forefinger of the left hand, and direct them towards the positions they are to occupy in the *coiffure*. Wave as before, holding the iron a little on the incline, so that the waves fall nicely round the head and join in with the waves at the sides.

WAVED COIFFURE.—The waving finished, pass the comb through the hair right round; then take the whole of it in the left hand at a suitable distance from the head, in order to avoid pulling it, or taking out the undulations, as the hair should remain as fluffy as possible. The front hair should be combed back in accord with the shape of the *coiffure* to be produced; and the same with the side hair. Then with the right hand slightly twist the hair to make a Grecian or Anacreon bow. For a chignon, a bunch of light curls can be added, the hair on the top of the head being combed backwards.

With short hair, instead of twisting it or making the Grecian knot, the ends should be curled, an india-rubber ring serving as a bind, and the hair being passed through it. This leaves the hair very fluffy, and admits of its being brought forward, or on to the sides, as may be required.

The ends of the hair should be curled over the finger, and form a very light chignon.

CHAPTER X.

WATER-MADE COIFFURE.

THE water-made *coiffure* was very fashionable during the latter part of the Empire. There are still ladies who have the flat water or indented curls arranged over

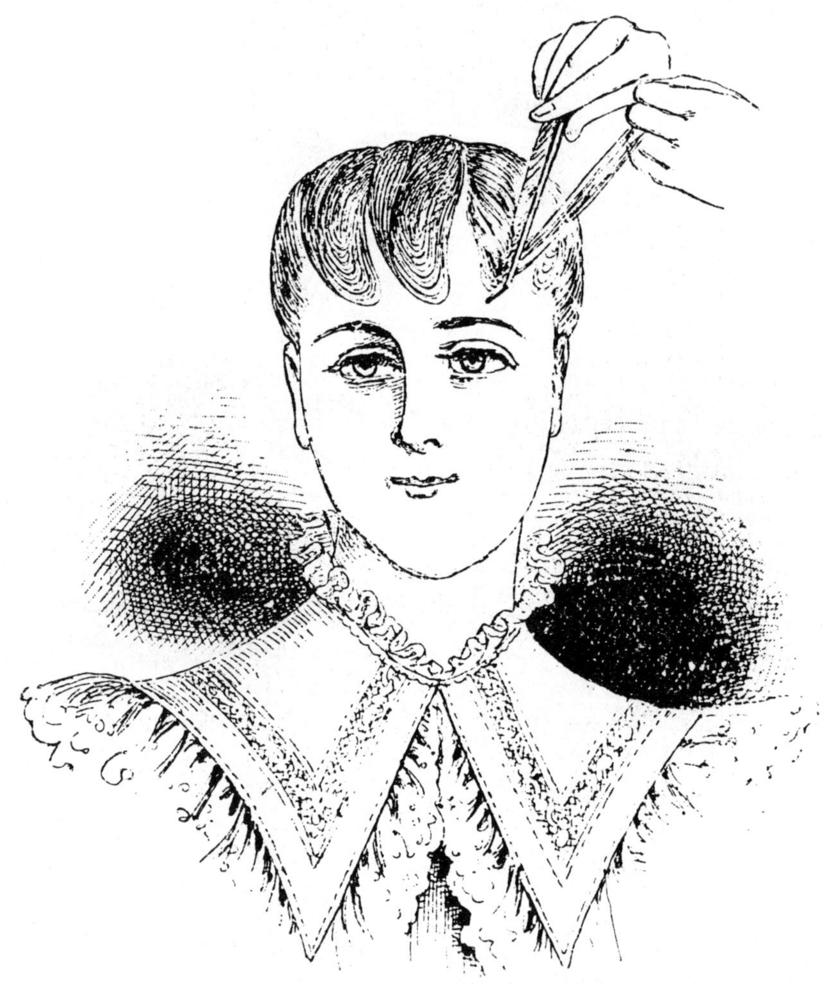

WATER-MADE INDENTED CURLS.

the forehead or on the top. The style suits ladies with dark hair.

FLAT WATER OR INDENTED CURLS.—To make these the hair is thrown back; pomade is rubbed in and then moistened with water, to which a few drops of spirit have

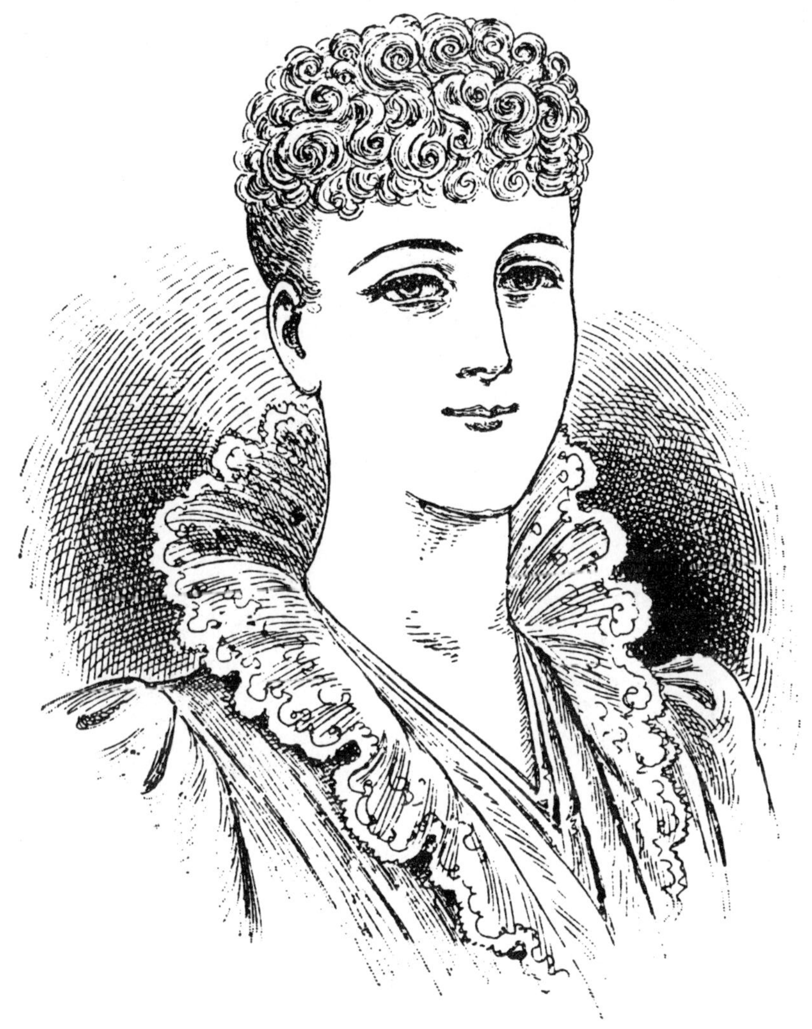

WATER-MADE CURL COIFFURE.

been added, after which the hair is carefully smoothed down. With the first tooth of the fine part of the comb a parting is made, commencing at the forehead. Take the hair on the fine part of the comb forward, and with the forefinger of the left hand keep the piece in place, while the right hand shapes the flat curl on tooth, finishing with a single hair. The first curl is made alongside the ear, and the others follow as shown in sketch.

In order to make a water curl *coiffure* (style Pompadour) the hair is fastened at the back ; but a fairly large piece is kept in front, going from temple to temple. This is rubbed with pomade, moistened and smoothed down evenly. The hair is then thrown well back, the points are taken with the left hand, and with the fine teeth of the comb the hair is brought forward.

In this way waves are formed one on the other, and give the impression of a *coiffure* of natural curls. The curls may be kept well flattened by placing a sufficiently broad ribbon over them, and the ends being held while the remainder is being finished.

CHAPTER XI

STUDY IN HAIRDRESSING.

IN the preceding chapters, we have described as clearly as possible the first and elementary operations which the artist is called upon to perform in dressing a lady's hair. We have explained how to make loops, bows, knots, twists, curls, waves, &c., &c.—and to have acquired thus much is certainly something ; but more than this is required from a good hairdresser. To dress a lady's hair is an art, and, notwithstanding his technical skill, the hairdresser can never succeed unless he possesses artistic taste, and love for the beautiful. The hairdresser should always keep himself informed of the latest fashions ; he should be able to judge what shape to give to a *coiffure ;* he should study the profile, and arrange the head-dress so that it blends with the features, is becoming, and enhances the looks of the client. For this purpose, besides possessing technical knowledge, the *coiffeur* should know the position of his client and the style of garments to be worn. It will easily be understood that, given two clients of equal beauty, the one of spare and the other of ample bodily proportions, differently arranged *coiffures* are required. These are delicate points, but in the exercise of his art the hairdresser has to understand them. Before beginning the dressing the hairdresser should take in the outline of his client—shape of the head, breast, waist, and the approximate age. A *coiffure* should not be made hap-hazard. Before combing the hair the profile should be studied, and corresponding to it the head-dress should be executed either forward or backwards. Of course, a *coiffure* is differently arranged for a client with a round face than one with an oval face ; if the client is of short stature, the dressing should add to it. For a round head, the high and pointed *coiffure* is indispensable. Artists, both in marble and of the brush, invariably make it a great point that the *coiffure*, the shape of the head, the build, and the toilets of their sitters, should form a harmonious whole. A well-shaped head may always be dressed forward, more or less ; further, the height of the forehead and the size of the nose are important items to consider. A forward *coiffure* makes the features recede, and *vice versâ*. For a person with very regular features these precautions are not necessary—let the *coiffure* be composed of curls or bandeaux, and it will always be becoming so long as the client is not too old,—in which case, of course, the effects of the march of time will call for attention.

CHAPTER XII

Young Ladies' Coiffures.

OF these *coiffures* there is an infinite variety ; but those falling down the back are unquestionably the most becoming, no matter if curled, plaited, creoled, or in the

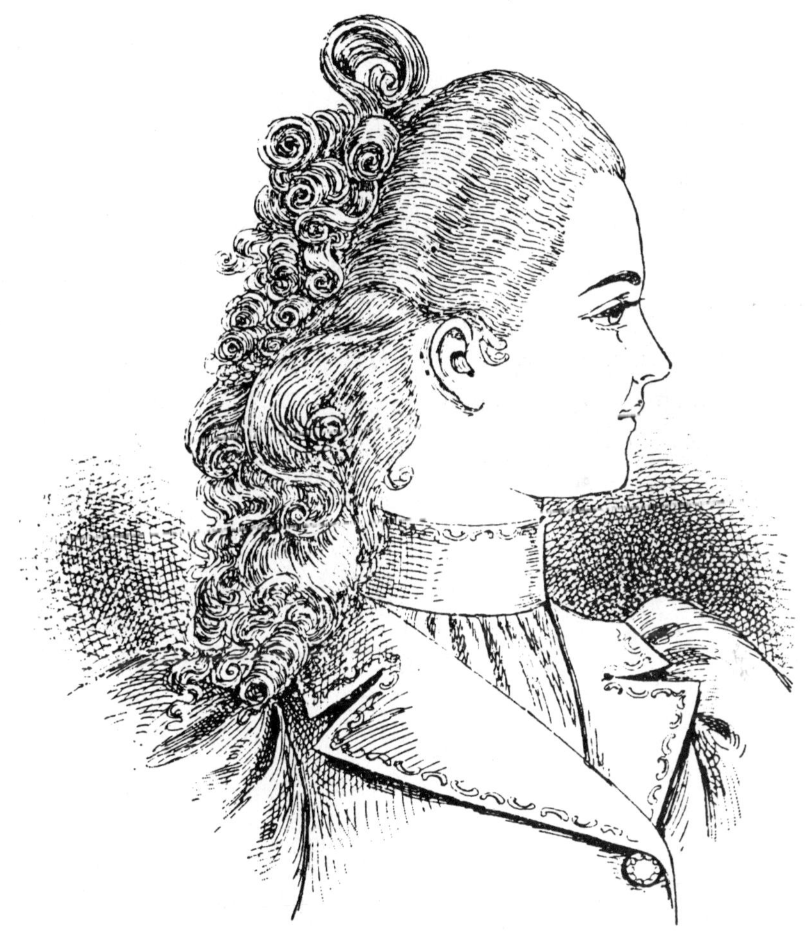

CURLED COIFFURE.

shape of a Catogan. The front hair is generally combed back, and forms a Pompadour puff. With tall young ladies, who require a raised *coiffure*, the hairdresser should take care not to obliterate their youthful appearance by dressing their hair as if they were full grown. To this end the head-dresses should be very simple and light, no matter

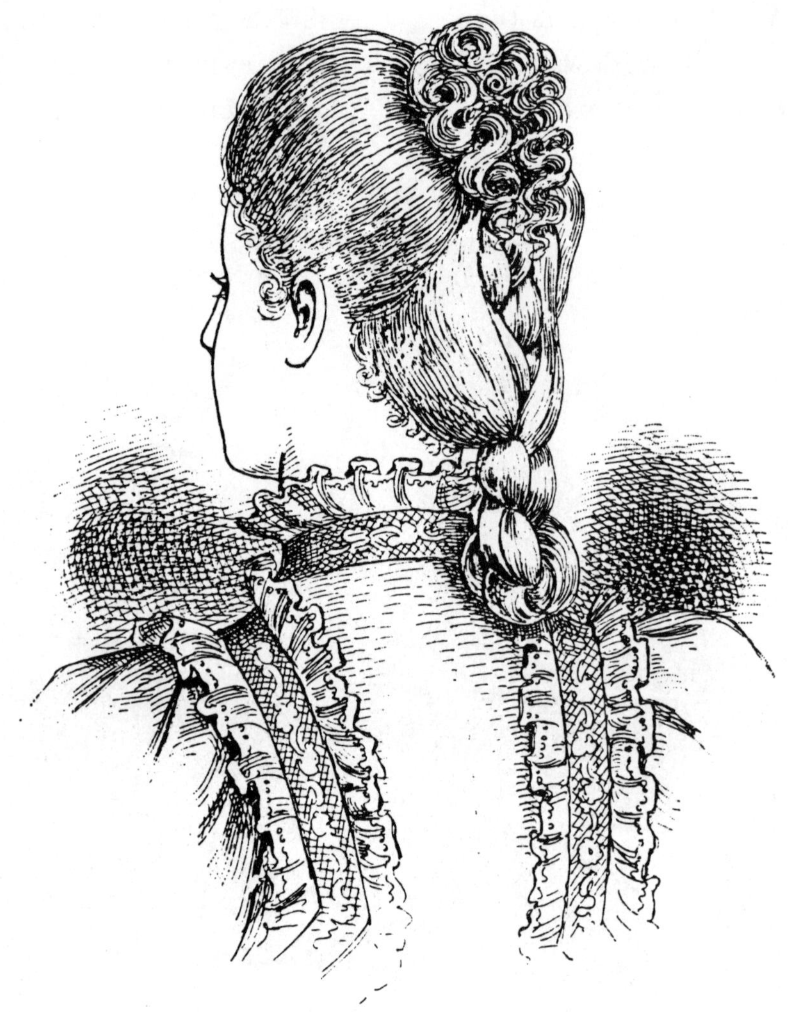

CATOGAN PLAIT COIFFURE.

whether the style be a Watteau (a few loops and the neck hair combed up), or of the present day (fluffy hair and a simple bow on the top of the head).

CURLED COIFFURE.—Make a cross-parting from ear to ear; fasten the hair on the top of the head, comb it up carefully in Pompadour style, and, if necessary, over a frizzett. Then put the hair in curl paper, and let the curls fall carelessly over the shoulders.

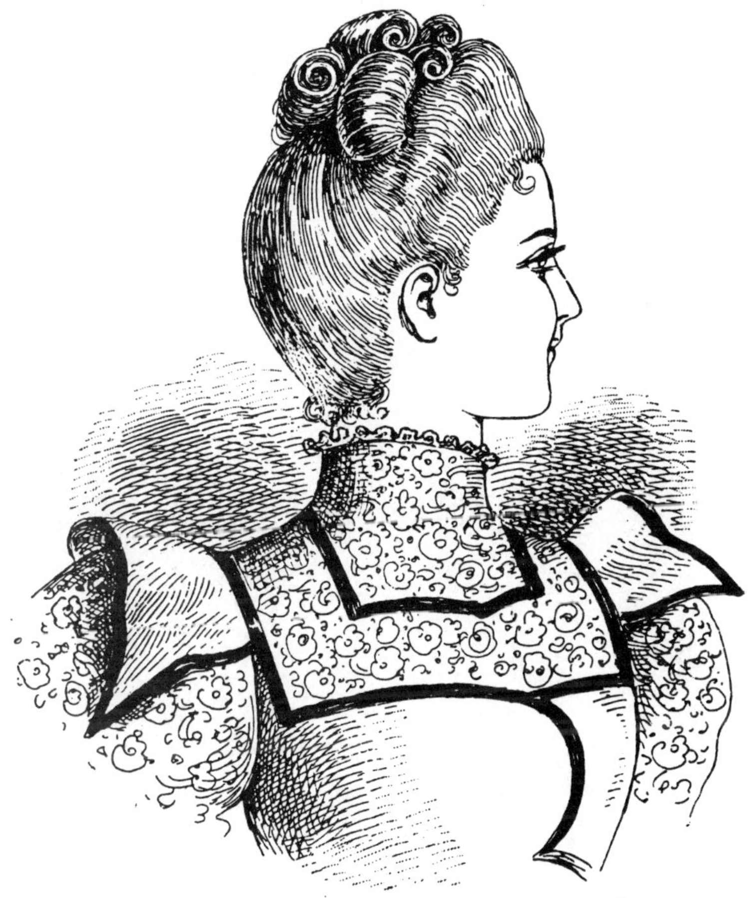

NECK COIFFURE (WATTEAU STYLE).

With fastened hair a bow may be arranged on the top of the head; or instead of being frizzed it can be arranged in spiral form.

THE PLAITED CATOGAN COIFFURE.—Make a cross-parting; comb up the hair in front and let it slightly bulge;

fasten it with a brooch on the top, rather backwards ; plait it, and lift the end of the plait underneath up to the nape of the neck, then pass the end of the plait between the rings ; curl the points, and form a bunch of curls on the

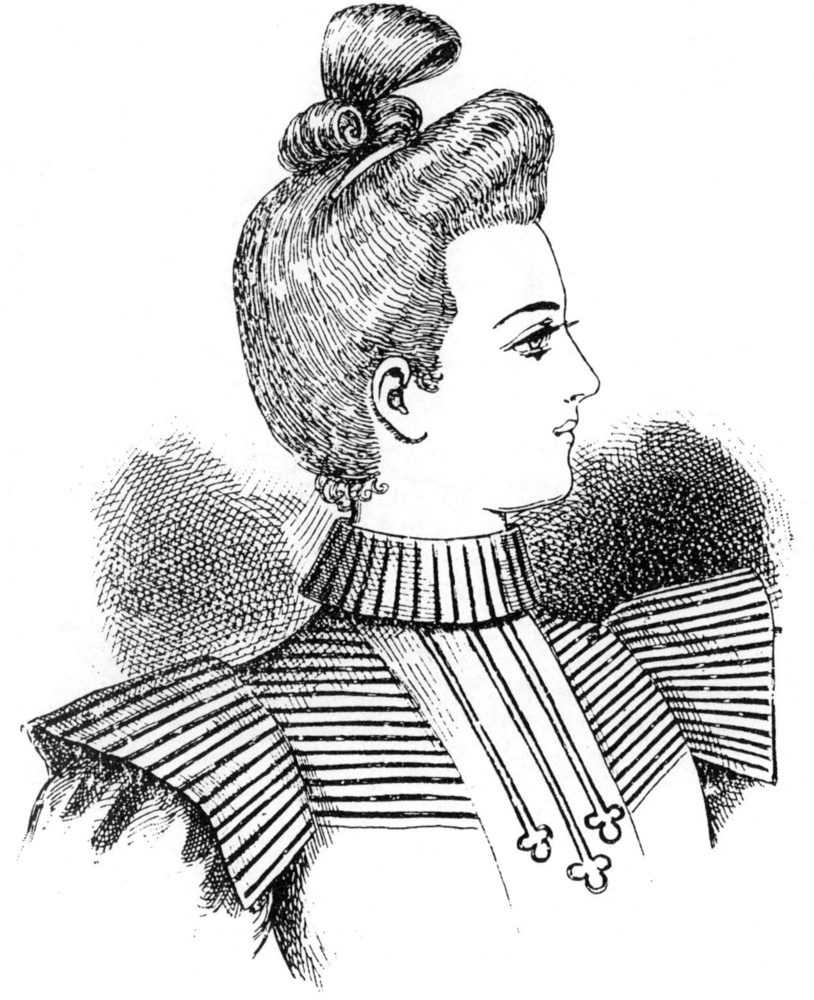

COIFFURE OF THE PRESENT TIME.

top of the head.   Should the hair be too short for a plait, a Catogan should be made, folded up inwards and tied with a ribbon.

H IGH C OIFFURE (Watteau style).—The cross-parting being made and the hair fastened, comb up the side hair in Pompadour fashion, and pin to the fastening ; with the hair of the fastening arrange a few curls on the top of the head ; pin up the neck hair and comb it up, and with the ends make a few curls ; give them a nice shape, and finish the *coiffure* with very light ringlets over the temples.

C OIFFURE FOR THE P RESENT T IME.—Lift up the whole of the hair very high and well forward. Twist it some distance from the roots, so as to leave the part near the head bulgy ; make an Apollo loop on the top, and by a half-turn of the hand push the front portion well forward, so that it stands out in front and at the sides. A single undulation right round the head can be made ; but waving has a tendency to make young ladies look older than they are. With this *coiffure* side-combs are generally worn : they keep the whole together and accentuate the style.

CHAPTER XIII.

LADIES' COIFFURES.

LADIES *coiffures* vary still more than those of young ladies, and their originator is that amiable, but capricious fairy, " Fashion." Every year she changes her style regularly. But we find also, that in consequence of an association of ideas, often inexplicable, if not from a desire for novelty and feminine coquetry, fashion is radically changed with each political or literary evolution. Hardly ever does an important event occur without bringing in its train more or less happy variations in the toilet and *coiffure* of the gentle sex.

In the time of royalty, the Queen and Court ladies set the fashion, of which they were the recognised and undisputed arbiters; in our more democratic times, it is the Theatre which has inherited this influence. The stars of the stage, more often than not, now promulgate new creations in the toilet and the *coiffure*.

Towards the end of the Empire, and in the early days of the Republic, ladies in general wore the hair falling down, and this necessitated the use of a large variety of postiche, in the shape of chignons—some being plaited, twisted, curled, or waved—which at the present time have almost entirely disappeared with the introduction of the Diana, the Grecian, and the waved *coiffures*. These latter have freed the necks of ladies, and to-day they wear the hair combed up high, resembling the styles of the First Empire and 1830.

Many of the fair sex, as a result of continuous waving, have a quantity of short hair. For this reason, the hair should be curled with the iron, and arranged in slight marteau curls of the Louis XV. style and tiny ringlets over the forehead, or even right round the head. In the

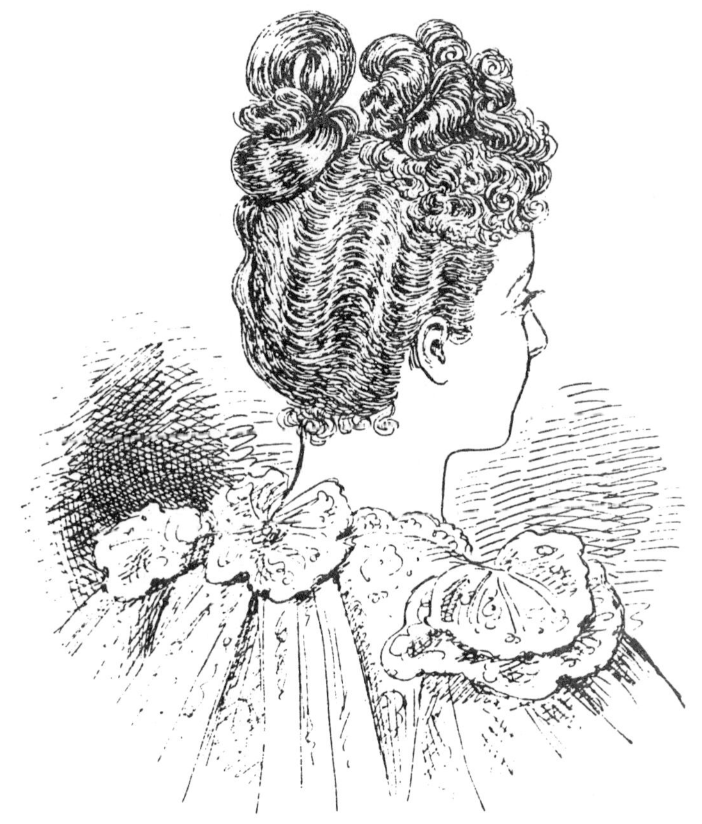

COIFFURE PUFF, LOUIS XV.

latest styles the neck hair is brought to the top of the head, and with the points a rather high loop, or bows, are made. The front hair should be left very fluffy, especially in the case of young ladies.

DESCRIPTIONS OF COIFFURES.

COIFFURE PUFF, LOUIS XV.—For this dressing, the hair right round the head has to be waved, and that on the forehead curled with the iron.   Take the whole of the hair

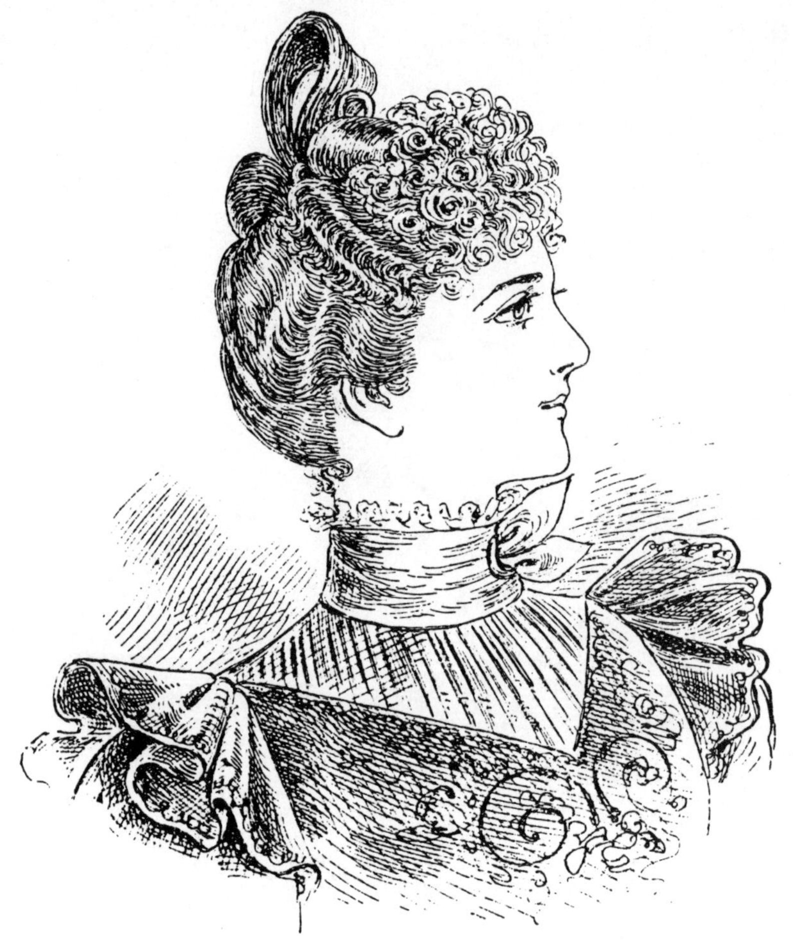

COIFFURE WITH PUFF AND SIDE PARTING.

straight from the roots to the top, and add a piece of 28-inch hair with curled points, which will serve for a soft bow on the top of the head, the ends of the natural hair being twisted round it.   The fringe should be arranged as stated. This style is elegant in its simplicity, and is suitable particularly for young ladies.

COIFFURE WITH PUFF AND SIDE PARTING.—To commence with, make a side parting and a cross parting; divide the back hair into two pieces, upper and lower;

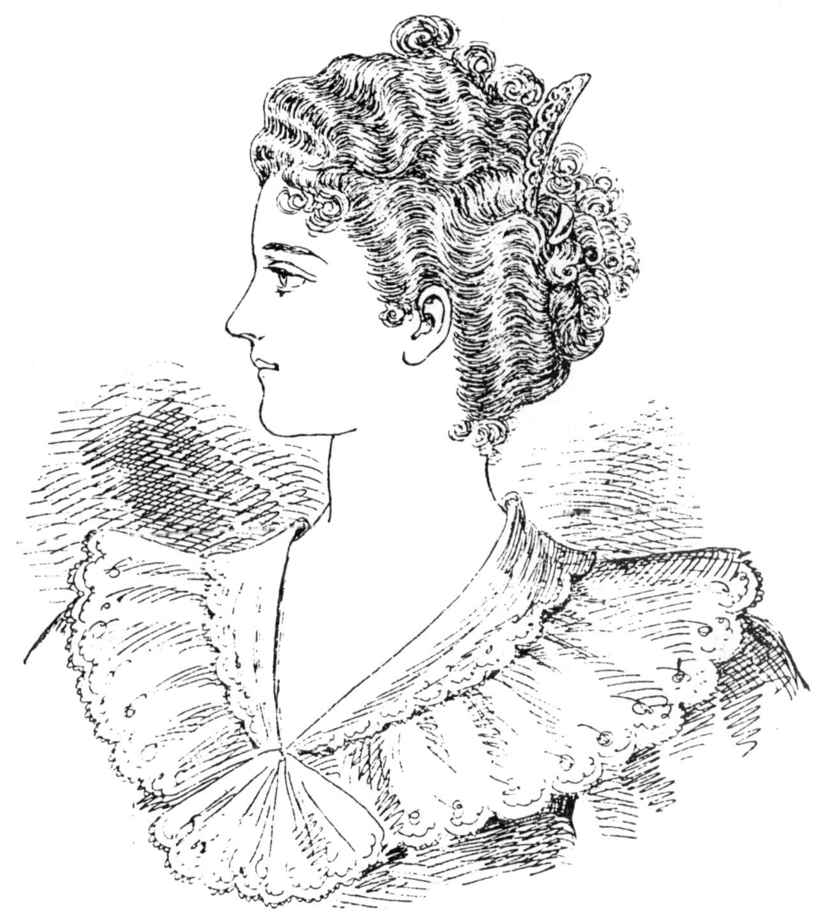

RAISED WAVED COIFFURE.

fasten the upper piece on the top of the head, and let the lower piece fall down. Wave the hair at the sides slantingly over the temples, and curl the front hair with the iron in a light fringe. Lift up the side hair and pin it to the fastening on the top. With the piece of hair fastened on the top make a straight loop with the hand raised, and with the ends of the side hair arrange two marteau rolls in front of the loop. Finish by taking up the lower piece

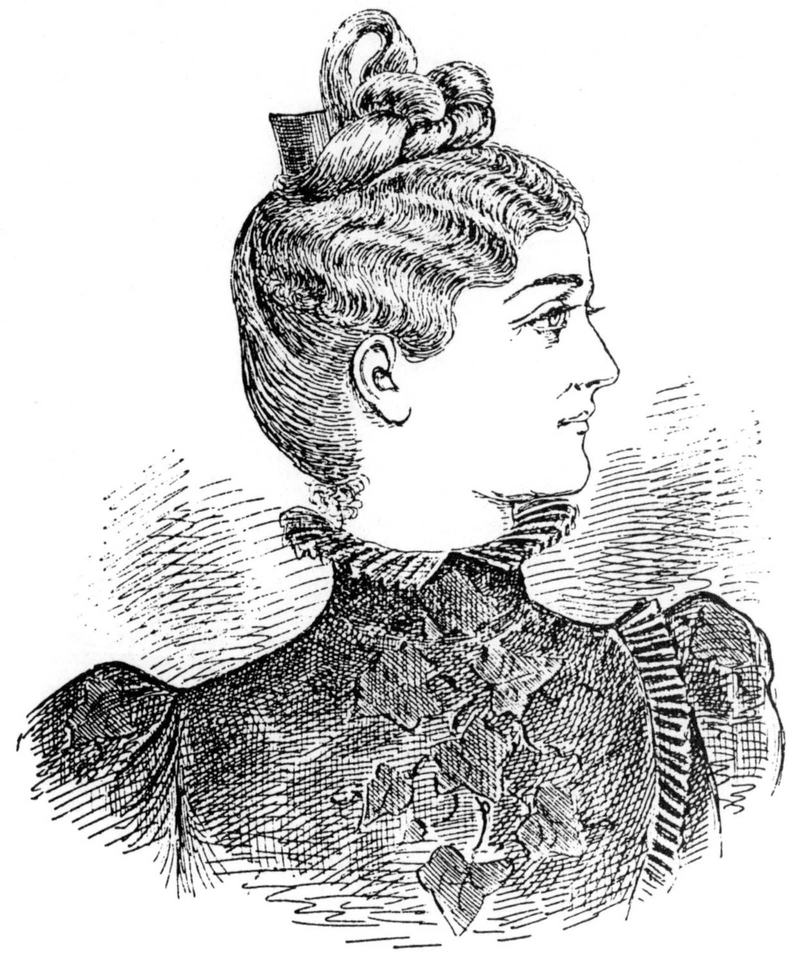

WAVED BANDEAUX COIFFURE.

straight from the roots, and twist the ends in ribbon shape round the loop.

RAISED WAVED COIFFURE.—Wave the hair right round the head; twist it loosely, and fasten on the top rather backwards, reserving the hair between the temples for a puff in front. Place a comb frizzett in position, and comb the hair over it Marie-Antoinette style. The chignon consists of light, spiral curls, as shown in engraving. Over the temples some very light curls are arranged in Louis XV. style, and a fancy comb can be placed behind to finish the *coiffure*.

COIFFURE OF WAVED BANDEAU.—This is suitable for ladies of a certain age, since it permits the hiding of bare places, which are so often found on the top of the head. Having made the middle parting, and waved the bandeaux in large waves, either on pin or with iron, the hair on the neck should be parted off and the remainder fastened on the top; then the bandeaux should be pinned to the fastening, together with a two-branch plait of about 28 inches. Each branch serves to make a Gordian Knot on each side, and they are joined at the middle of the parting. Comb up the back hair and make a loop with the points. For ornament use an Empire comb.

CHAPTER XIV.

ORNAMENTS FOR THE COIFFURE.

THE women of all ages—ever graceful daughters of Eve—have ornamented their hair with flowers, feathers, ribbons, lace, gauze, &c., as well as variously shaped ornaments, pins, combs, diadems, &c., from the very simplest to the most elaborate and artistic, made of precious metals and studded with gems of every kind. To properly choose and place these ornaments, the hair-dresser requires both experience and taste. The position, the colours, the shapes must be in harmony, not only with the *coiffure* itself, but with the features, and the complexion of the lady and her toilet in general. The colours should suit the age, the shade of the hair, &c. The slightest want of harmony and uniformity may ruin the effect of the best *coiffure*. General rule : Everything that is striking and vivacious produces a very good effect on dark hair, and brightens a dark complexion ; red and yellow are the colours for brunettes. For blondes, on the contrary, rose colour and pale blue harmonize best with the whiteness of the complexion and the colour of the hair. For brunettes, therefore, deep red, cherry, light yellow, chamois, crimson, black and gold colours ; for blondes, rose, light blue, green, lilac, violet and azure blue. For ladies with brown hair and of dark complexion, the colours for brunettes are suitable ; those with fresh rosy complexions should wear the colours for blondes. The positions for combs, pins and jewels are generally indicated by their shape. Diadem ornaments become persons of regular features ; but under all circumstances the hairdresser should use ornaments to

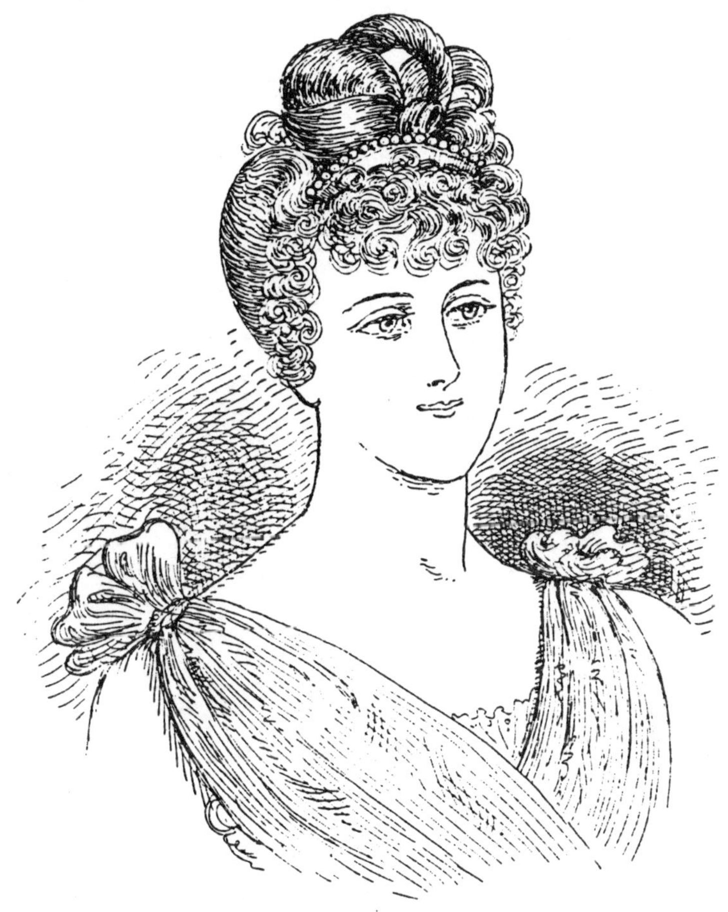

COIFFURE WITH EMPIRE DIADEM COMB.

enhance the appearance of the head-dress he has executed. With the client sitting before the glass, the hairdresser is able to judge of the effect produced, and to see if, and how far, the head-dress harmonizes with the features, toilet, expression, &c. It is a delicate matter to decide, as the best executed *coiffure* may be entirely disfigured by inartistic ornamentation ; it entirely depends on the skill and good taste of the hairdresser.

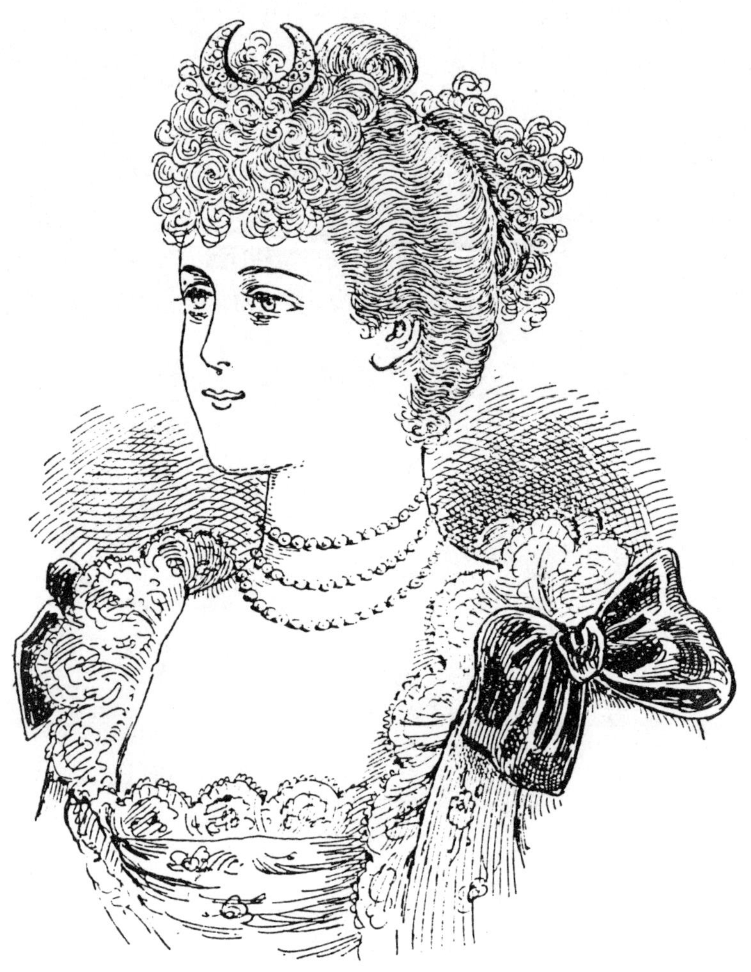

COIFFURE WITH CRESCENT ORNAMENT.

COIFFURE WITH EMPIRE DIADEM COMB.—Fringe the front hair right round with the small iron, or put in paper ; fasten on the top, and make the bandeau in raised Pompadour style. With the points form a bow on each side, rather forward. The neck hair should then be lifted up, postiche added, and interlaced with the bows. The fringe should be nicely arranged in conformity with the face; and the diadem comb should be placed as shown in the engraving.

COIFFURE WITH CRESCENT ORNAMENT.—Wave the hair right round the head in large waves; arrange a light fringe in front in a bunch (or utilize an artificial fringe); make a fastening on the top; and with the fastened hair make a loop with the hand raised. Gather the back hair loosely, and pin it at the back in chignon form; and round the middle of this wind a 10-in. marteau curl. The crescent can then be placed as shown in the engraving.

To Use Ribbon.

To interlace the ribbon with the hair, a shell needle is used; bows are made in the same way as milliners make them for hats, and sometimes the ribbon is arranged into a bunch of loops, stiffened with wire to keep the loops up straight; at other times a hairpin is run through the ends of the ribbon and the loops obtained are used as ornaments.

THE RIBBON LOOP COIFFURE.—Make a side parting in front and then the cross partings; lift up the bandeau (on the right side higher than the left); pin them to the fastening; with the points make bows at the sides; comb up the neck hair and form a very high loop with raised hand; curl the ends of the hair, and arrange the ringlets round the soft bows of hair. Fix the ribbon ornament at the side as shown in the sketch.

COIFFURE WITH INTERLACED RIBBON.—Wave the hair slightly right round; make a fastening on the top; lift up the whole of the hair loosely and pin it firmly to the fastening ; add a piece of hair with curled ends, and twist it round the bandeau. With the hair of the fastening

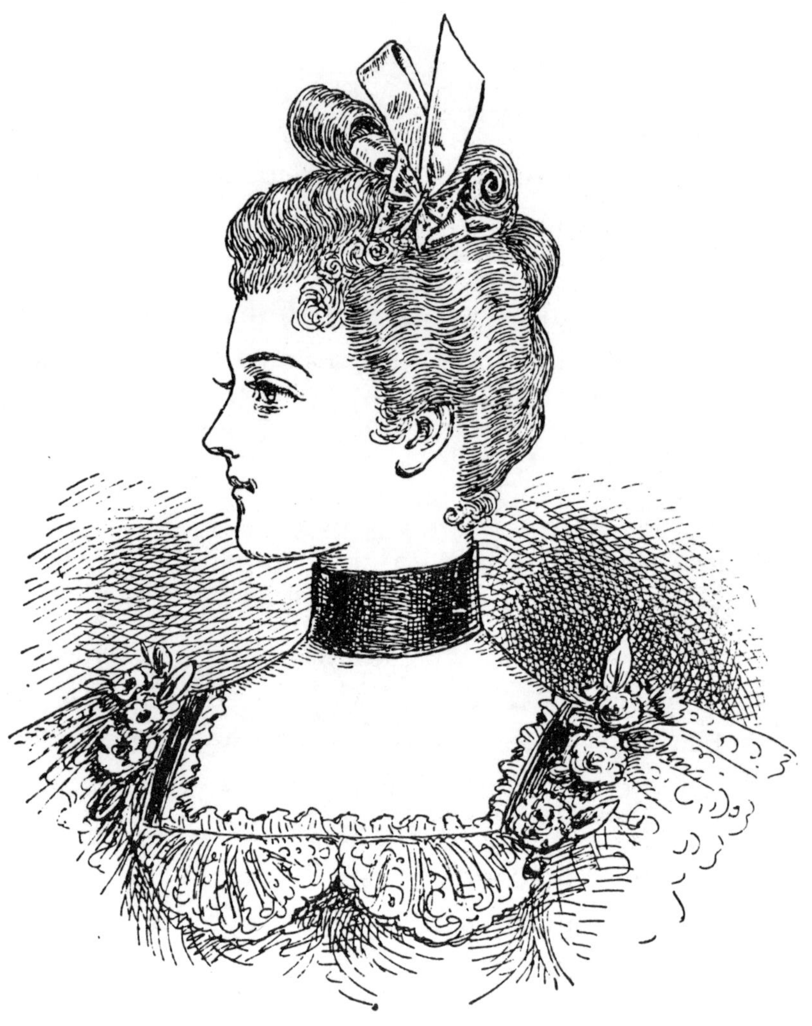

THE RIBBON-LOOP COIFFURE.

make a few bows with raised hand to form the chignon ; with the ends of the additional piece arrange some light curls ; dress the front fringe in light ringlets ; with a shell needle

draw the ribbon through the *coiffure* right round the head
and the twisted piece, as shown in the design ; draw out

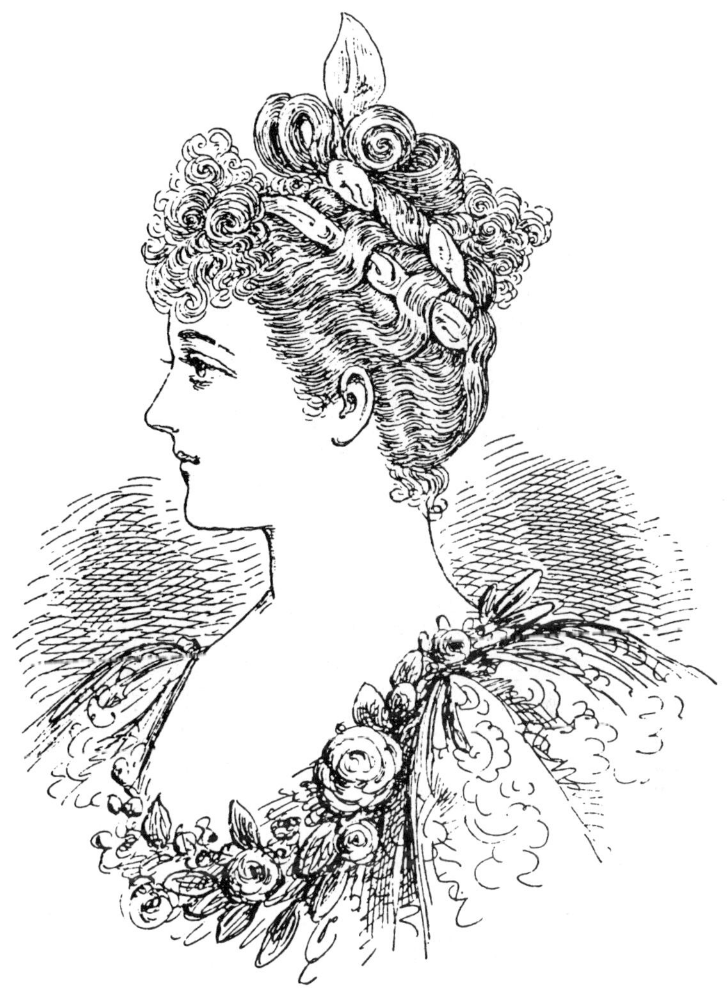

COIFFURE WITH INTERLACED RIBBON.

the end of the ribbon on the top and work it in the shape
of a leaf, or any other suitable form.

CHAPTER XV.

WEDDING COIFFURES.

THE wedding *coiffure*, as in fact *coiffures* for all grand ceremonies, does not differ much from the soirée dressing, since it has to follow the fashion of the day. Anything eccentric must, of course, be avoided—that is the hairdresser's business. For several reasons the *coiffure* should be as near as possible to the style in which the client usually wears her hair. The ornamentation of the wedding head-dress is simple, consisting as it does of orange blossom, mounted in wreath fashion, or placed in bunches at the side, and a veil of tulle or lace. The veil is arranged in different styles, such as the Jewish, the Spanish, the Renaissance and others.

WEDDING COIFFURE.

The hair is done in large waves right round the head; a cross parting is made, and the hair in front parted in the middle between the temples (a fairly thick piece being reserved); a fastening is made, and the hair taken up in the shape of a very high loop on the top. With the front hair a forward bulging puff should be formed, the short hair being curled into a light fringe; after which the temple hair should be curled, and the wreath of orange flowers placed in position.

How to place the Veil, Jewish Style.

This style is most often seen on a bride. The white tulle veil (cream colour for a brunette) should be long enough and sufficiently large to cover the whole toilet. In front it should reach below the waist, and at the back to

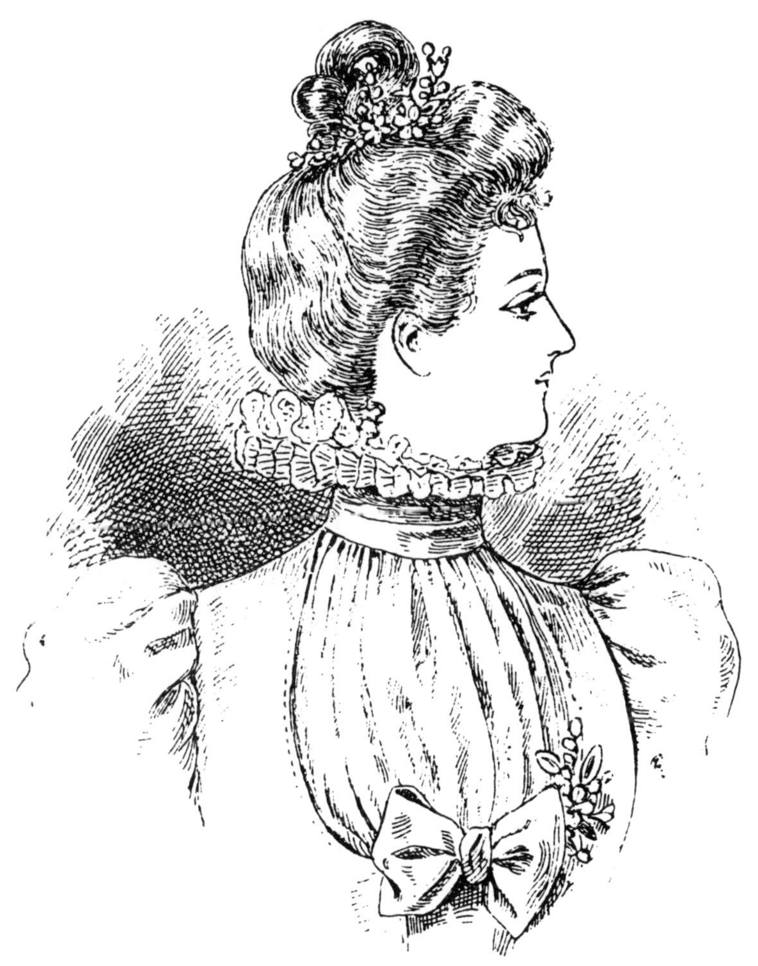

WEDDING COIFFURE.

the end of the train. The veil should be placed in position when the *coiffure* (wreath of orange blossoms included) is finished, and just before the departure of the

bride for the ceremony. The veil is arranged as follows :—
It is first unfolded over the arms of the hairdresser, and
he, standing behind the bride, who is also standing, places
the veil on the top of the head, allowing for sufficient in

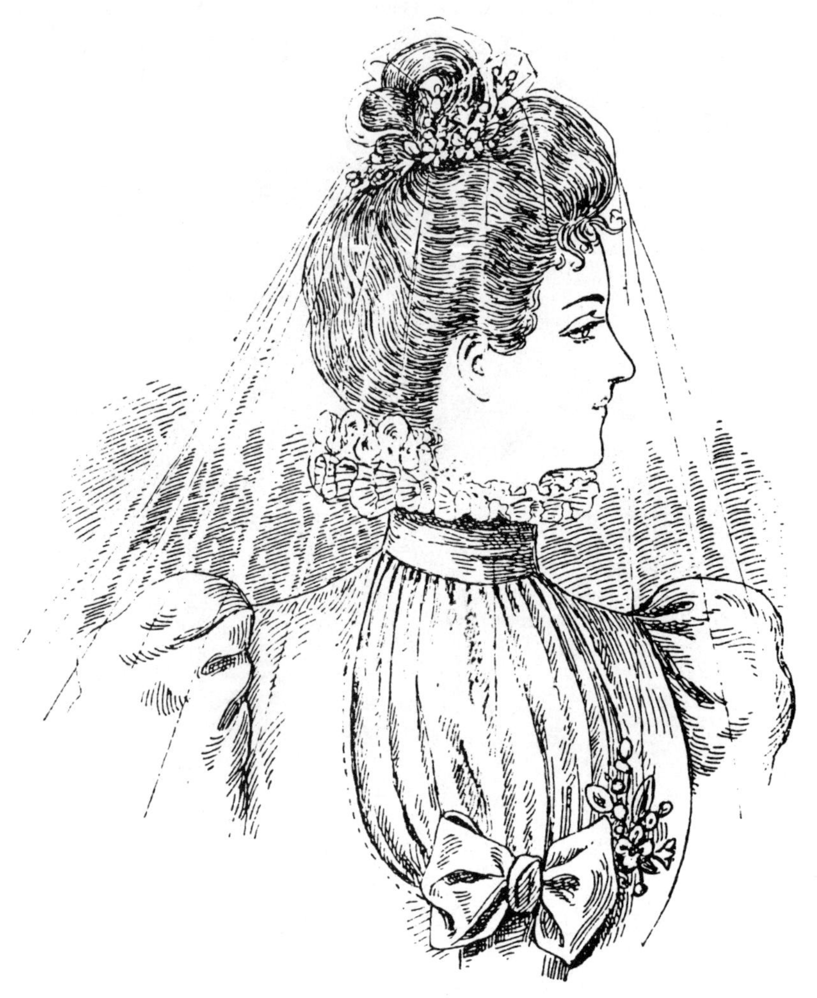

JEWISH STYLE OF VEIL.

front to fall over the face down to below the waist. It is put
in folds on the top of the head, and the folds, pinned so as
to form a kind of *aureole* (halo), should reach down to the
end of the train. No fold must be seen in front over the

face. Then the four corners of the veil are rounded off with the scissors, and where the veil reaches beyond the train it is cut right round at the end of the train.

THE SPANISH STYLE OF VEIL.

When the hairdresser arranges a lace veil in Mantilla

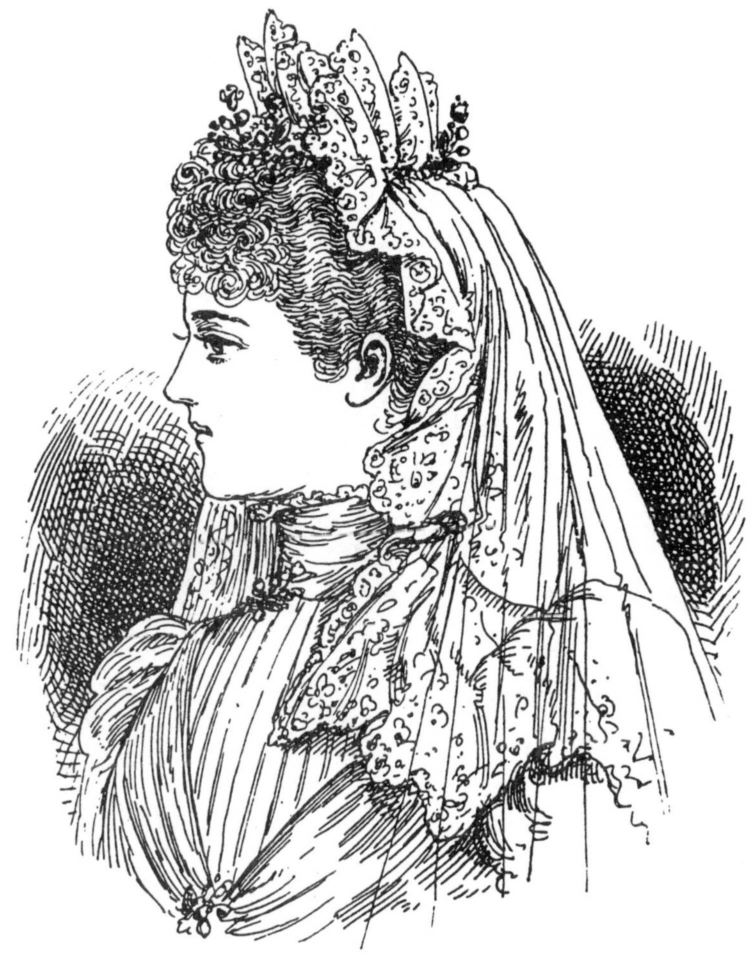

SPANISH STYLE OF VEIL.

style, or, where the lace is too thick, the face is left uncovered. The veil should be pinned to the *coiffure*, allowing the orange blossom to be seen as much as possible. Altogether, it should assume the graceful form which

Spanish ladies know so well how to give to their mantilla. The folds of the lace fall over the shoulders.

THE "RENAISSANCE" VEIL.—Having pinned the veil on the *coiffure* behind the wreath, rather high loops of lace

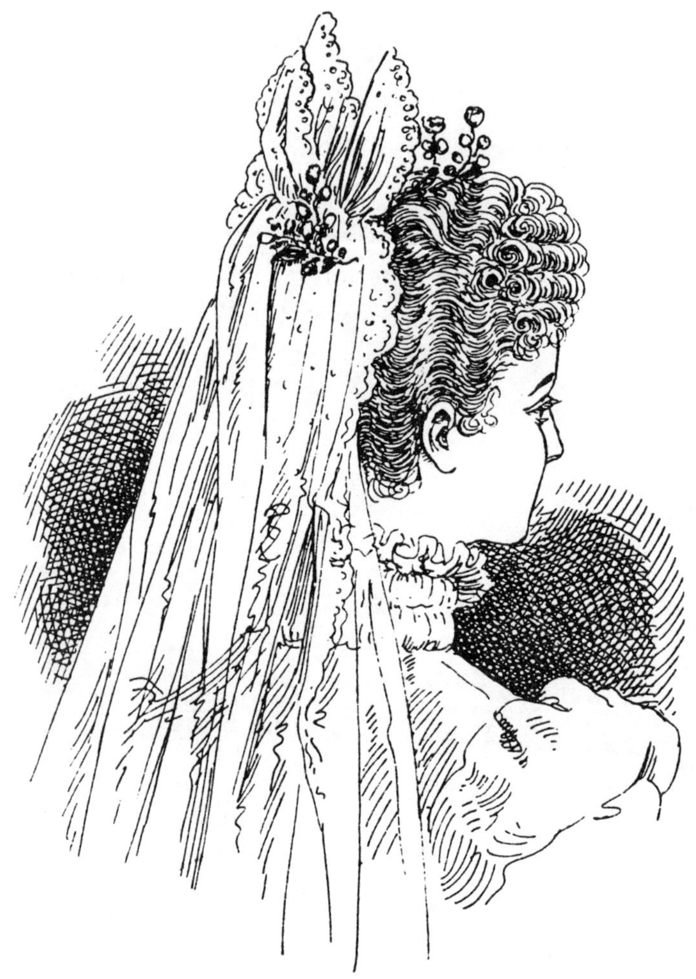

RENAISSANCE STYLE OF VEIL.

are arranged, and a sprig of orange blossom is fastened at the foot of the loops at the back. The veil is allowed to fall down at the back in the graceful fashion of the court mantle.

CHAPTER XVI.

BALL AND SOIRÉE COIFFURES.

COIFFURES for balls and soirées must always be elegantly executed and prettily ornamented, in harmony with the remainder of the toilet. The hairdresser should know, before commencing, what ornaments are to be worn, since, by their kind, form, and location, he has to be guided. For instance, if a wreath of flowers has to be used, he must study which position will be most suitable for it, and in which it will gracefully and artistically adapt itself to the features. For a sprig of flowers at the side, he should have previously arranged the place in the *coiffure*; the same with diamonds and precious ornaments in general; these should be firmly fastened on account of their weight, and should be displayed as much as possible.

On occasions of public balls and official receptions, hairdressers are so much pressed for time, having only a few hours to satisfy quite a number of clients, that it becomes a matter of necessity that the work is done quickly. In these cases ladies appreciate the work of a hairdresser when executed with precision, rapidity, and quick decision in the choice of ornaments. It is an excellent proof of his professional skill, taste, and experience in the art of hairdressing The positions of the flowers vary according to their shape, colour, and mounts; and this is equally the case with almost all ornaments. The Bacchante wreath is placed high on the forehead;

the Ceres requires a regulaɪ pose ; a Mary-Stuart crown is placed backwards on the crown ; a Chaperone is placed at

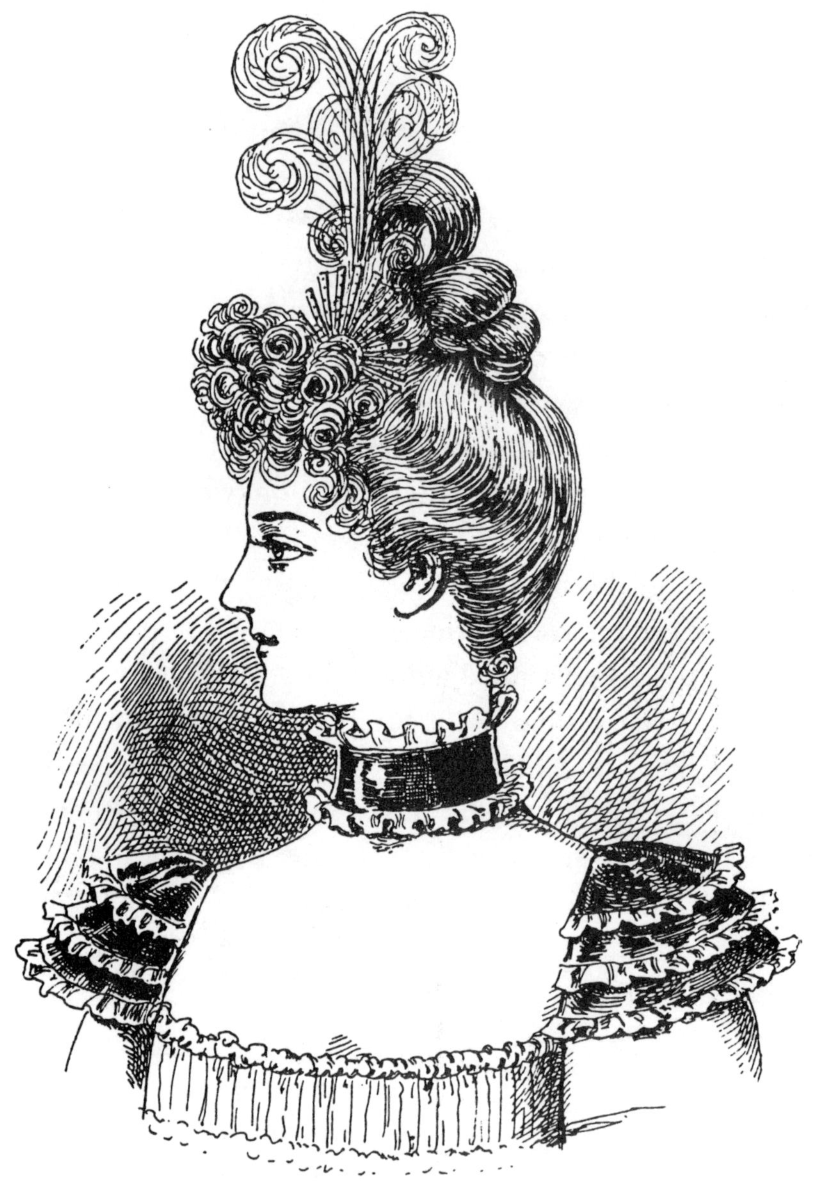

YOUNG LADY'S BALL COIFFURE.

the side, dividing the *coiffure* in two ; fancy garlands and detached flowers, having nothing specially characteristic about them, can be arranged in many different ways—and here the inspiration of the artist can alone serve him.

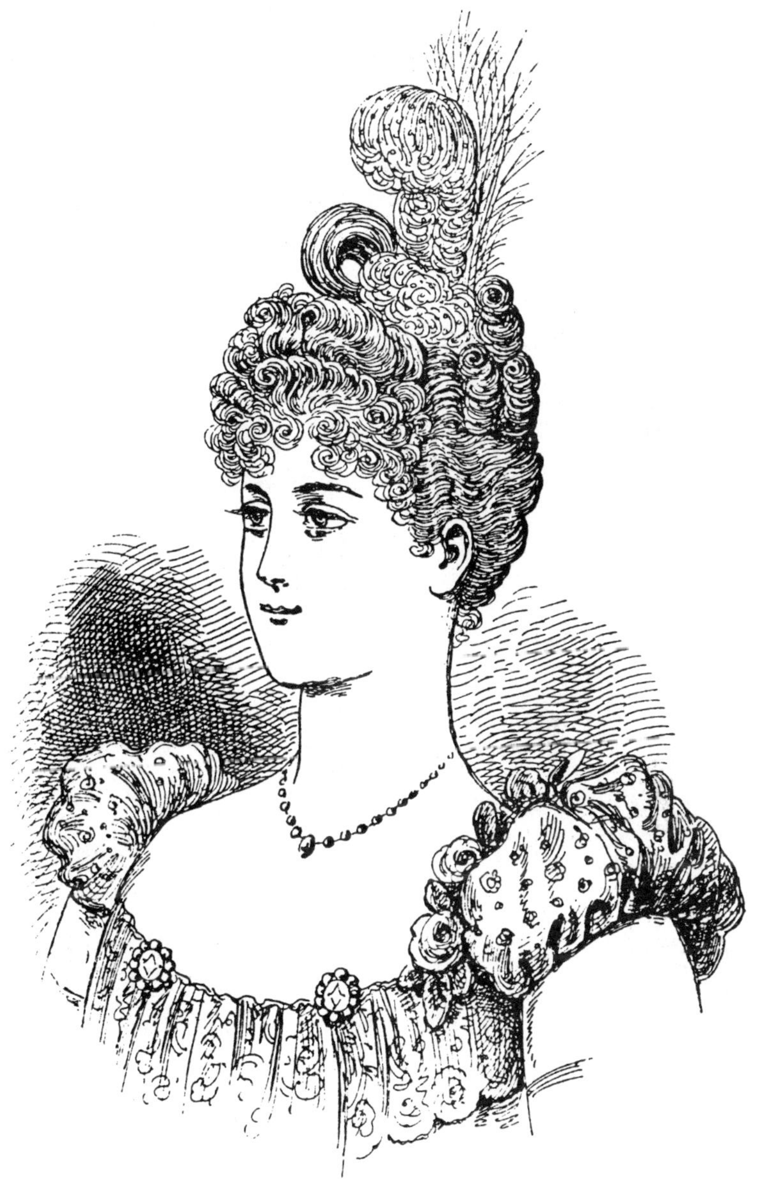

OPERA COIFFURE FOR YOUNG MARRIED LADY.

Aigrettes and plumes are treated like detached flowers. When a hairdresser knows how to arrange flowers, he can build up any style of *coiffure*, so long as it harmonizes with the ornaments.

With cashmere or gauze for ornament, the former should be arranged in graceful folds, the latter in light plaits; the colours should be suitably selected to harmonize with the features. The *coiffure* should be of a size proportionate to the head, no matter whether a turban or baret has to be formed, or simply gauze is employed.

DESCRIPTIONS OF SOIRÉE COIFFURES.

No. 1.—Young lady's ball *coiffure :* The hair is waved right round the head in broad waves; for a fastening a small plait is made ; then the whole of the hair is lifted up, and an Apollo bow made with the loop very high ; the ends of the hair are twisted round it; the short front hair is made into a fringe and forms a bunch of curls resting on the forehead ; and the parting is arranged at the side. Ornaments : an aigrette of Paradise feathers and a row of pearls.

No. 2.—Opera *coiffure* for young married lady : The side hair is waved in broad waves ; the hair over the temples is done in light curls; the middle part is dressed in light puffs, style Louis XV. The whole of the hair is lifted up and an upright loop is placed rather forward. Add a few marteaux curls at each side, as shown in the engraving. Ornaments : a bunch of plumes, and an aigrette, with roses under.

No. 3.—Ladies' grand soirée *coiffure :* The side hair is waved, lifted up and made into a Grecian bow on the top backwards ; a 24-inch piece, mounted on a hairpin, is passed through the ring of the bow, twisted and made into an 8, to form the chignon, as engraving; the waved ends are allowed to fall down on the neck; the front hair is curled with a fine curling iron, and dressed Louis XV. style; and two marteaux curls are made on the top to

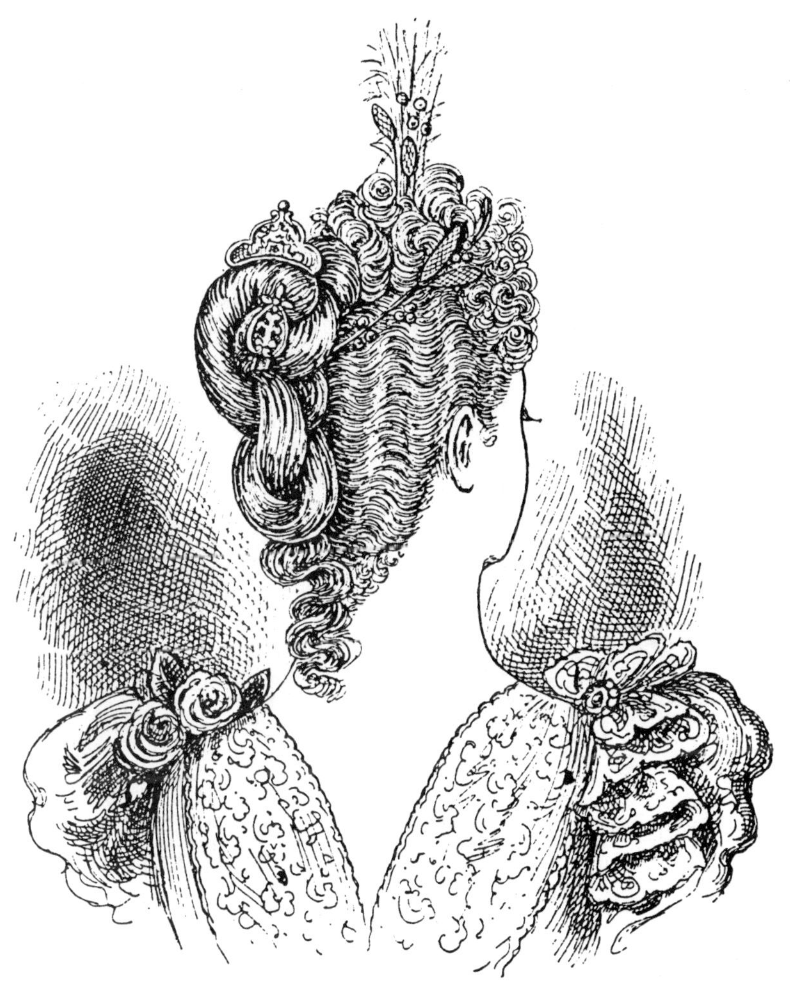

LADY'S GRAND SOIRÉE COIFFURE.

round off the *coiffure*. Ornaments: a wreath, the leaves studded with diamonds, aigrette in the middle, comb and fancy pin with diamonds.

No. 4.—Elderly lady's grand soirée *coiffure:* The bandeaux are waved on hairpins; a chignon in coil-shape is arranged at the back; the waved bandeaux are combed

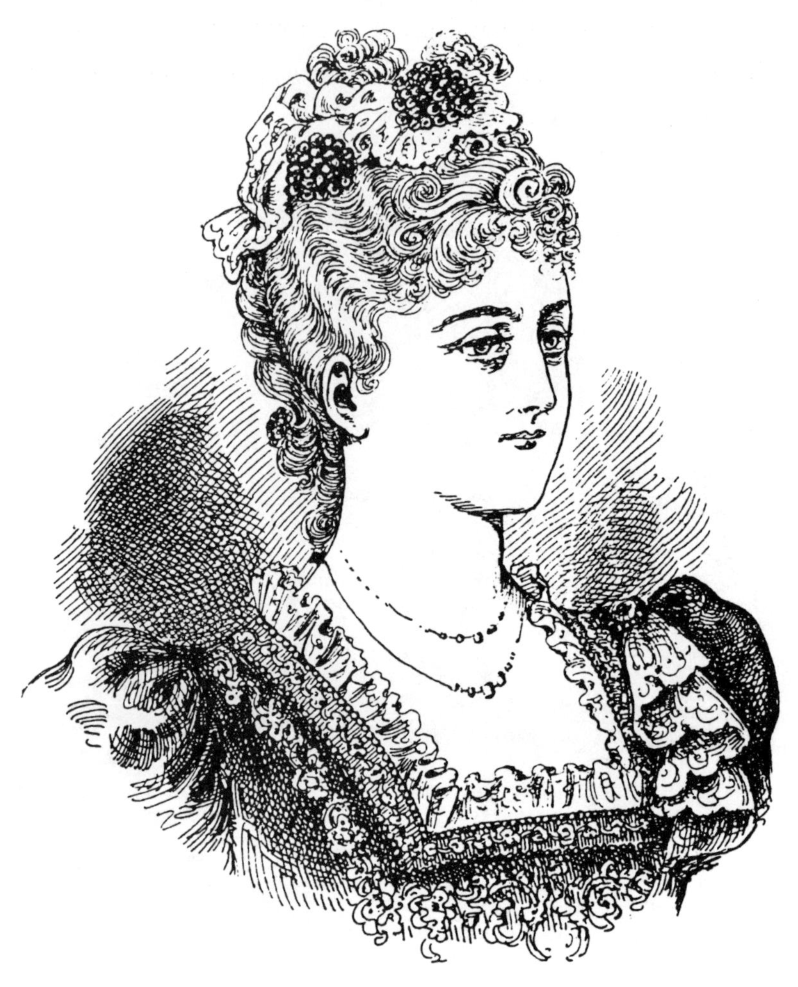

ELDERLY LADY'S COIFFURE.

over the temples, which they cover; the ends of the hair are twisted round the chignon; the front is dressed by combing up the hair in the middle and adding small curls to the temples, unless front postiche is required. On the top some slight marteaux-curls are added, the whole making a light *coiffure*, which yet hides any bare places on the crown, &c. Finally, place on either side of the middle parting a curl, as per engraving. Ornaments: a lace scarf of the form of a Louis XV. chaperon, fastened with fancy pins, ornamented with jet.

CHAPTER XVII.

Coiffures with Postiche.

THE greater number of *coiffures* require postiche in some form or another. It increases the volume of the natural hair; does away in certain cases with curling, and dissembles the colour of the hair, should it be necessary. It is indispensable where the head shows bare places, or where the natural hair is too short. Postiche, however, should always be very carefully adjusted, so that the effect is such as to deceive even a practised eye. The postiche most often employed, and which we shall call "classical postiche," comprises tails or switches, plaits, curls, marteaux, pin-curls, frizzetts, chignons, knotted fringes, transformations and wigs. All these, made to perfection, should be as light as possible. It is to the advantage of every hairdresser that he should be a good postiche-maker, or at least that he should know how it is made; he should know, also, how to properly take the measurements for it, especially where a wig or a transformation has to be supplied.

In the case of a wig, begin (1) to take the measure round the head; (2) from the forehead to the neck; (3) from ear to ear across the top; (4) from ear to ear across the forehead; (5) from temple to temple round the back. These five measurements correctly taken, suffice to construct a wig which will fit well. The hair to be knotted

must be of a length suitable for the lady's features, and to
obtain the perfect illusion of a natural head of hair.

COIFFURE WITH TRANSFORMATION.

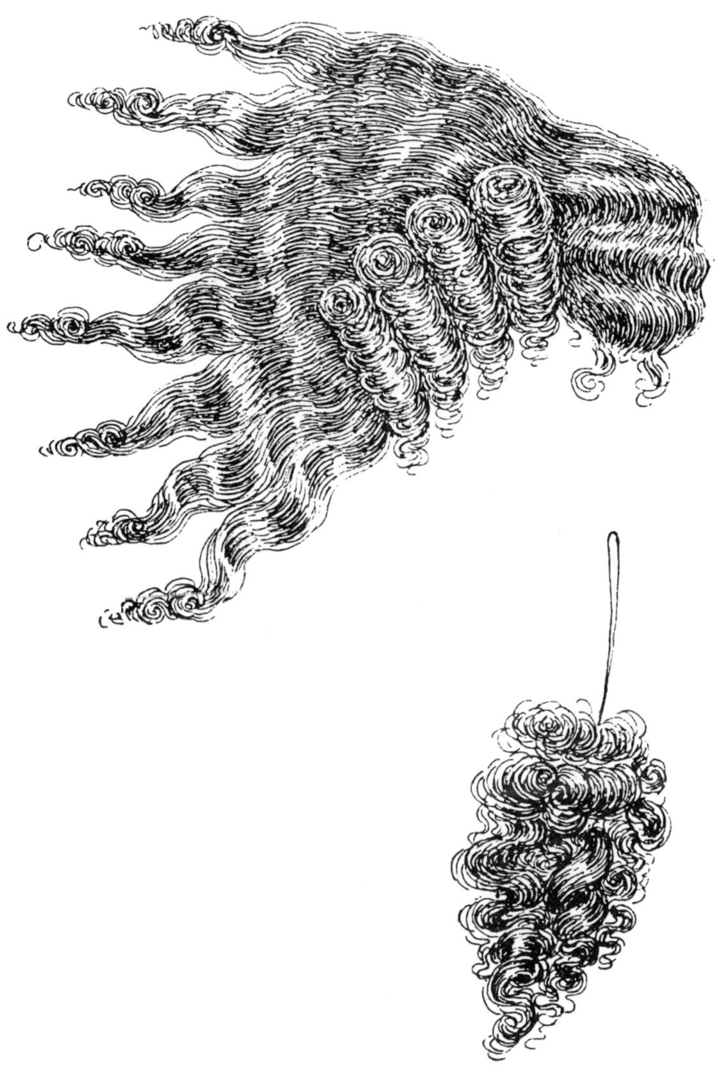

TRANSFORMATION POSTICHE.

For a transformation, it is sufficient to take the measure
round the head; but it is advisable to take it also across the

forehead and across the top. The front fringe being postiche on a small scale, or part of a wig, every hairdresser should be well up in the making of it.

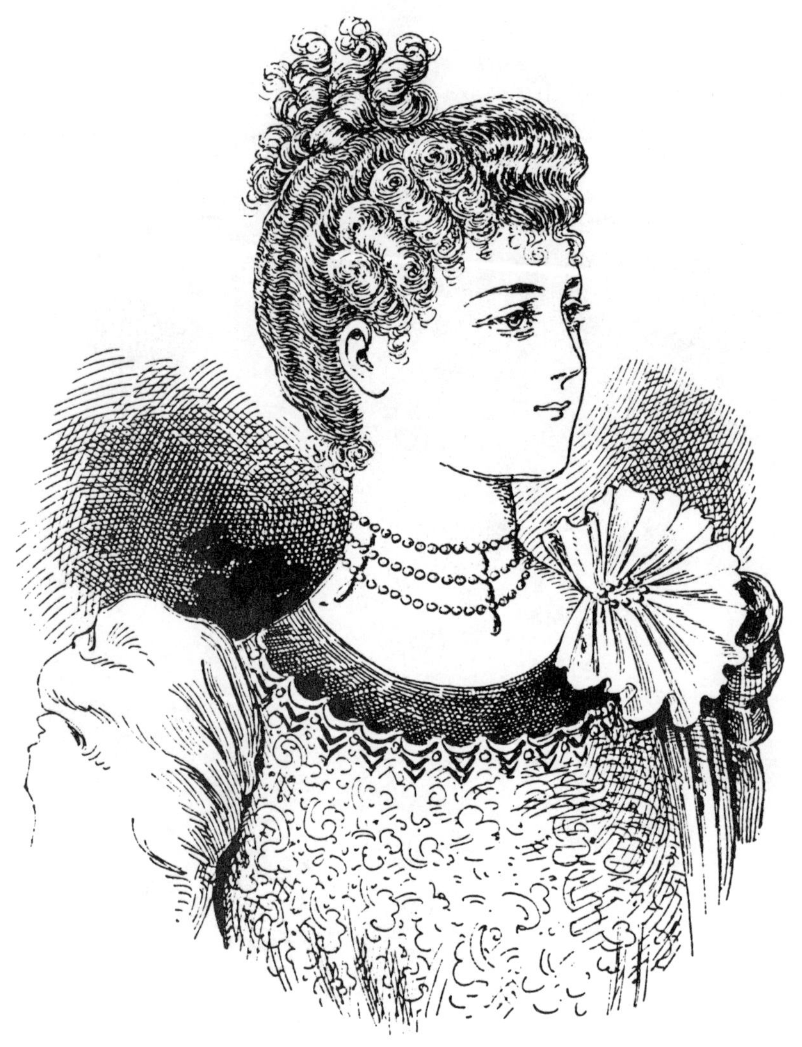

PIN CURL AND COIFFURE.

Comb up the whole of the natural hair; plait it or twist it on the top, so as to occupy as little space as possible; adjust the transformation, and firmly fasten it at the base of the neck. A chignon with curled ends should be arranged, and some pin curls added. The natural hair must not be seen at all.

WIG COIFFURE.

The natural hair is treated in the same way as before, and the wig is adjusted, while the two points of the wig, near

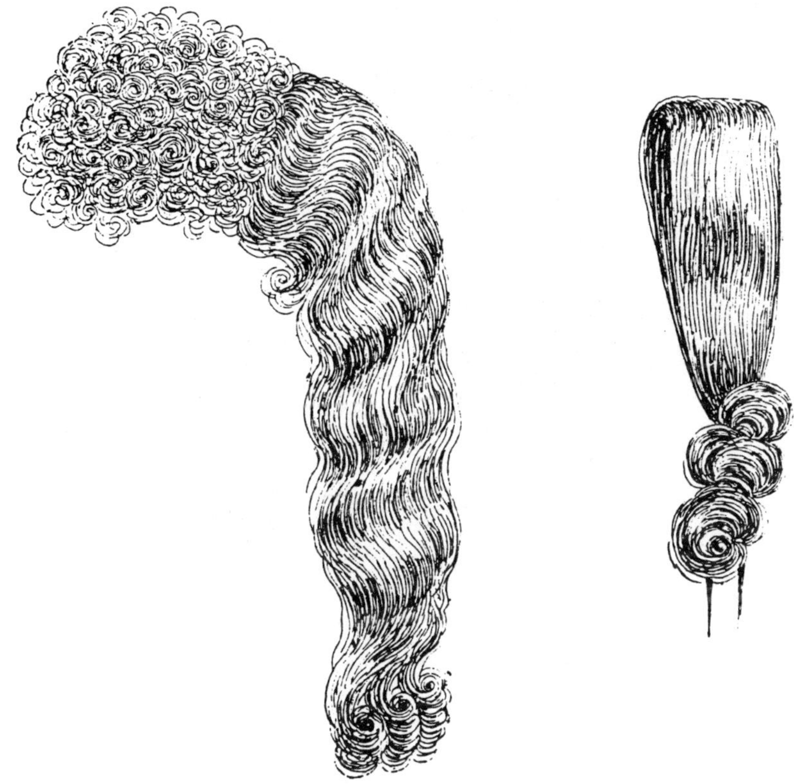

WIG AND LOOP, 1830.

the ears, are firmly held (if possible, by the client); the hairdresser then draws down the two sides over the neck, unless it is a wig open at the back. The *coiffure* is made as if with the natural hair, adding the necessary postiche, such as switches, marteaux, or even a chignon.   The dressing in the engraving is made with a loop, mounted on a pin, and two marteaux curls.

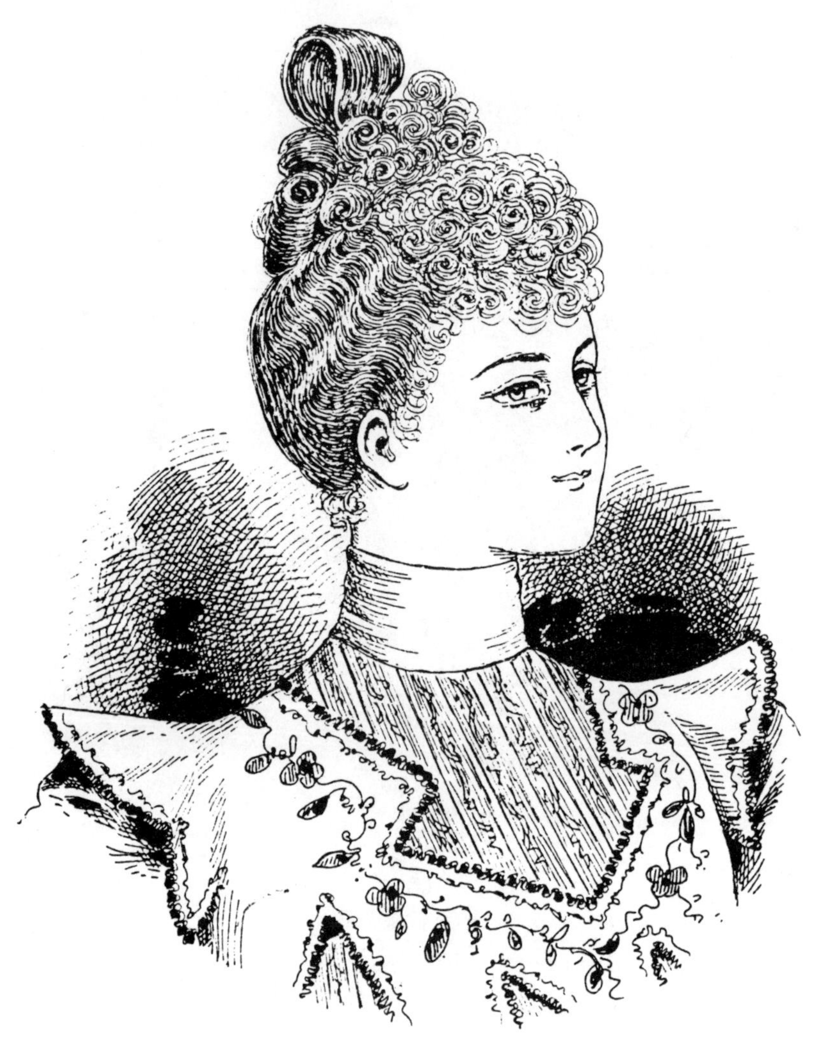

COIFFURE MADE WITH WIG.

CHAPTER XVIII.

POWDERED COIFFURES.

WHEN dressing a lady with light brown or blonde hair, hair-powder is very often used, either to obtain a lighter shade, an ash colour, or a more reddish tint. Sometimes grey hair has to be hidden, where the client objects to dyeing. For this purpose the hairdresser has to choose a powder giving the hair the requisite tint, and suitable to the complexion and expression of the client. The application of the powder—a not very difficult matter—should be carefully done with a puff all over before the hair is dressed, or else when the *coiffure* is completely finished. When, however, dressings with white powder are to be executed the case is different. These are the *coiffures* of the end of the last century, generally known under the names of powdered *coiffures*, Louis XV. and Louis XVI. For the execution of these, the hairdresser has to thoroughly study the styles, and must, besides, have artistic taste, as they are above all else artistic. The Louis XV. *coiffures* are exceedingly elegant in shape, comparatively small, but proportionate to the size of the head. The Louis XVI. dressings are of more original and majestic build, very large and voluminous all round ; often exaggerated, and out of all proportion to either the head or the build of the person. Although these styles

are not generally worn in our day, it is indispensable
that a hairdresser should have studied them, so as to be
able to reproduce them when required. They are often
wanted for soirées and fancy dress balls.

In order that the powder may adhere well to the hair,
the operator, before executing the *coiffure*, should make a
powder foundation : for this purpose he must well grease
the whole of the hair, and then powder it with the special
powder (poudre à poudrer) applied with a large puff. The
hair should be waved on hairpins right round the head,
and treated with the pinching-iron to ensure lightness. When
marteaux and curl-postiche is used with this *coiffure*, this
addition should be powdered in the same way as the
natural hair, and tightly curled before being dressed and
adjusted to the head-dress. All postiche should be ready
prepared before the dressing begins. The powder foundation of the natural hair should also be made some time
before the execution of the *coiffure*, so that the curls and
waves have time to get cool.

MAKING-UP.

White powdered *coiffures* entail the use of grease paints,
to render the complexion lighter, as without them the skin
would look darker by the effect of the white powder on the
hair. The face and shoulders should be treated, before
the dressing, either with liquid "blanc," applied with a
sponge, or "blanc-gras" (white grease), applied with
cotton wool; then "rouge de Jouvance" should be
applied on the cheeks underneath the eyes; the lips
should be painted carnation-red; eyebrows and lashes
blackened, to make the eyes sparkle; the ears should

be painted a rosy tint ; and finally some tiny black patches, of various shapes, should be stuck on in the

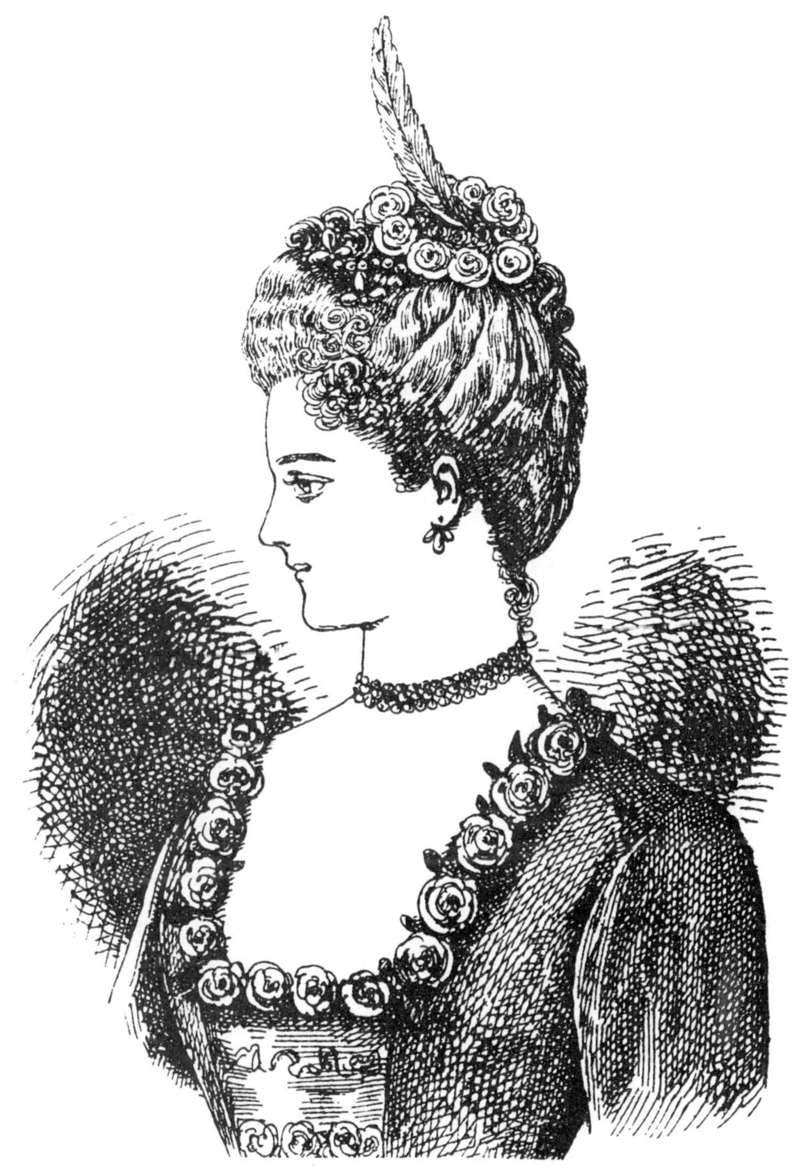

POWDERED COIFFURE, LOUIS XV.

fashion of the last century. This operation is a delicate one, and requires a certain amount of taste, since the object of the make-up is to give the client a younger and prettier appearance than before. If the hairdresser succeeds in this, his client is pleased, especially when the original features are somewhat homely.

POWDERED COIFFURE, STYLE LOUIS XV.—The powdered foundation made and the make-up finished, the execution of the *coiffure* is commenced by making a fastening on the top of the head backwards. The hair round this should be reserved for the *coiffure*, to a width of two inches all round the head. The hair is divided into pieces, and with them marteaux Louis XV. are made, the front hair being combed back and dressed. For making the marteaux, slightly crape the pieces above, twist them over the fingers and successively pin them to the fastening, commencing at the temple and continuing right round the head. The front hair is arranged in Pompadour puff fashion; tiny ringlets are made at the temples; with the points of the hair some light loops are formed, or marteaux curls are arranged. Then the white powder is applied by holding the puff in the right hand and beating it on the left, so that the hair gets evenly powdered all over. Ornaments : at the side a wreath of roses and a feather, with a diadem of pearls in fancy style in front.

COIFFURE MARQUISE, LOUIS XV.—The hair is combed up in Pompadour puff style and fastened on the top backwards. The back hair is loosely lifted up and secured with hairpins to the fastening; five marteaux are arranged on each side and firmly pinned to the head, the last being a curl-marteau, as shown in the engraving. To hide the ends of the hair a few light marteaux are arranged behind. The powder is then applied as in the previous *coiffure*.

Ornaments : a rose, surmounted by an aigrette of white feathers, placed at the side near the temple.

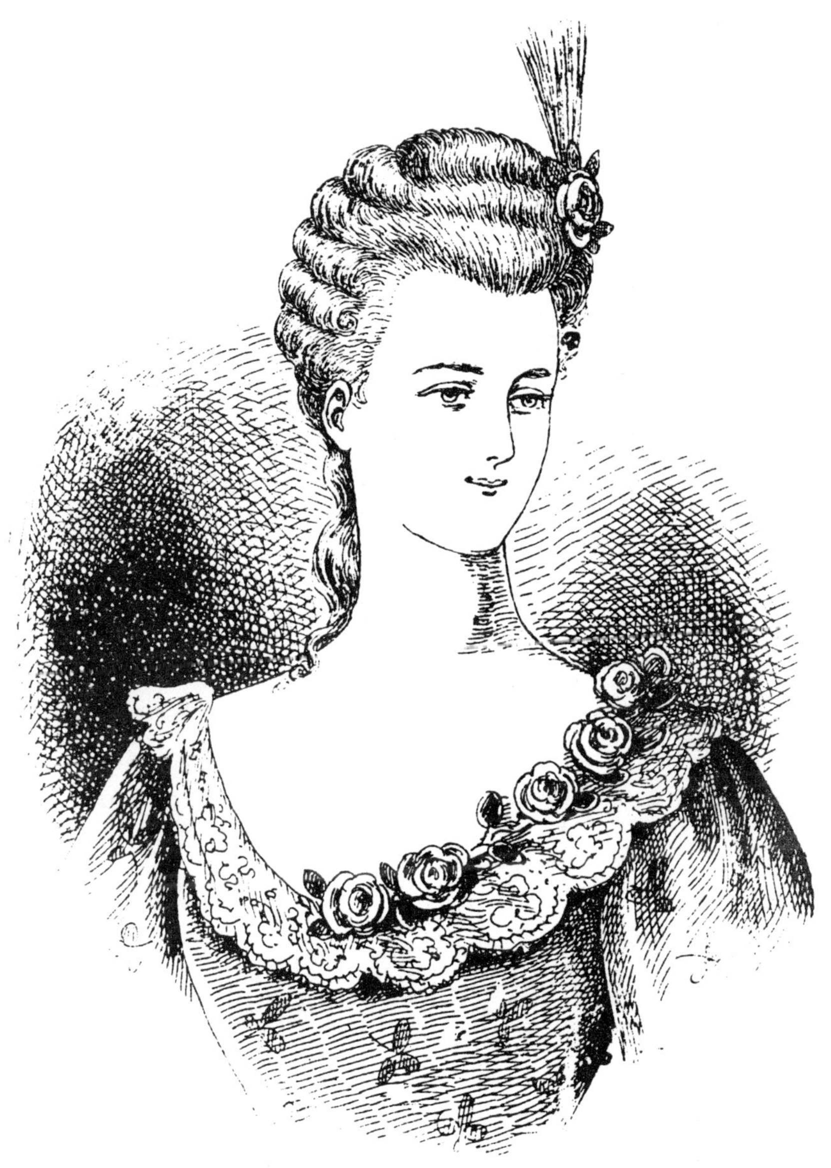

COIFFURE MARQUISE, LOUIS XV.

POWDERED COIFFURE, LOUIS XVI.—A cross parting is made and a fastening on the top backwards.   The hair is then combed over a rather large Louis XVI. frizzett. In making the powder foundation care should be taken to curl the hair and to put the ends of the front hair in curl-papers, so as to dress it in curl-marteaux. They are lightly

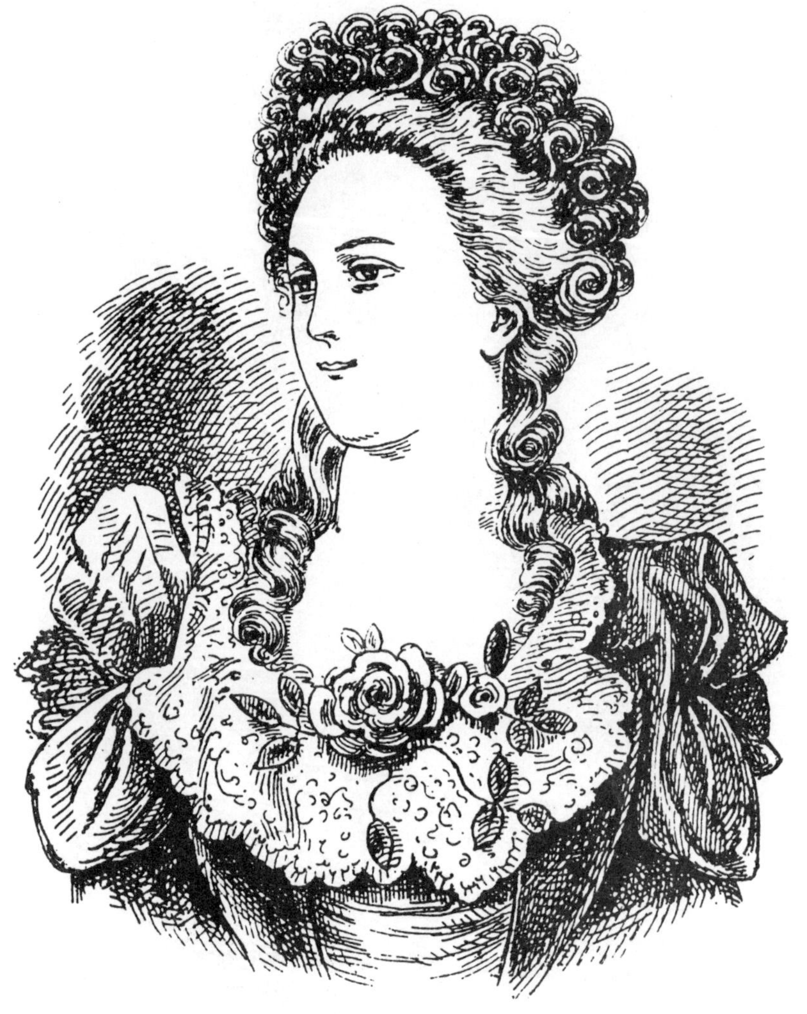

POWDERED COIFFURE, LOUIS XVI.

pinned backwards on the frizzett, and the artist should be careful to give them the shape shown in the engraving.

With the hair on the neck a Catogan loop is made, the

points being fastened at the top ; it is allowed to fall down between the shoulders ; a small bunch of marteaux-curls, Marie-Antoinette style, is arranged on both sides, and they

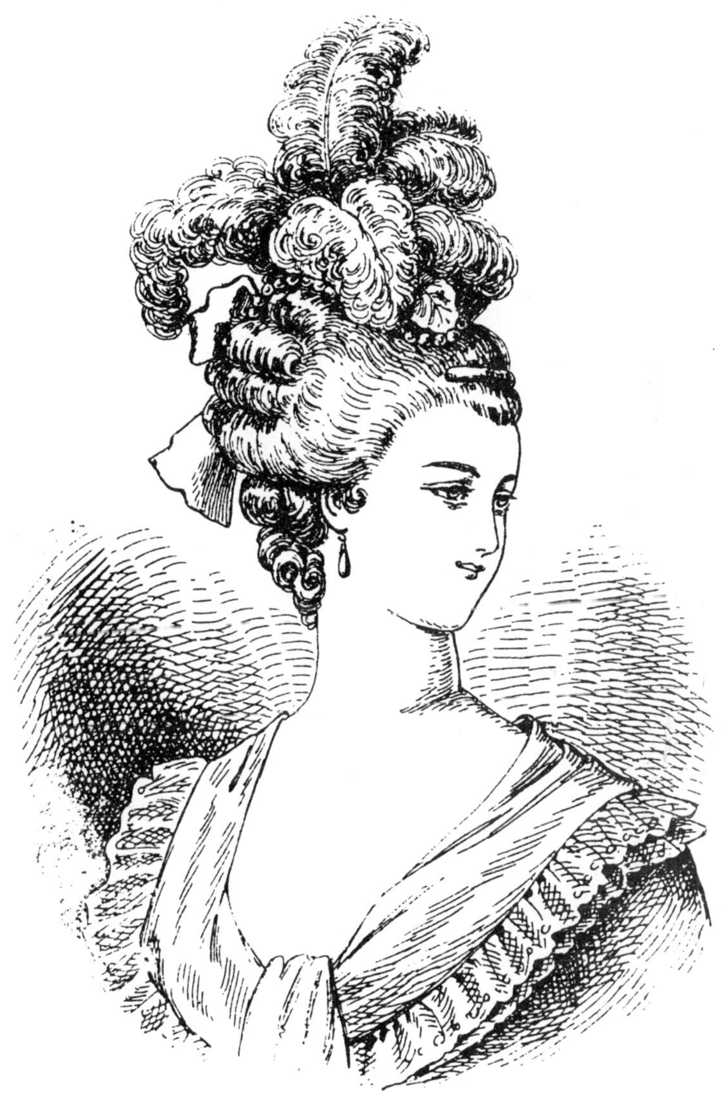

COIFFURE LOUIS XVI., WITH PLUMES.

fall down along the neck in front. The powder is then applied. Ornaments : a large ribbon bow underneath the Catogan.

Coiffure with Bunch of Plumes, Louis XVI.—A cross parting is made, the front hair is combed over a Louis XVI. frizzett, forming a Marie-Antoinette puff; the points of the hair are rolled over the fingers and form marteaux, which are fastened behind on the top; the neck hair is combed up, and with it a Catogan loop is made, which falls down at the back between the shoulders; it is fastened at the top. Marteaux-curls, Louis XVI. style, are placed on both sides near the ears. Ornaments: large bunch of ostrich feathers, ribbon bow, a comb with a plain narrow top, and a string of pearls, arranged as shown in the engraving.

M. CAMPBELL'S
IMPROVED FRENCH WIGS.

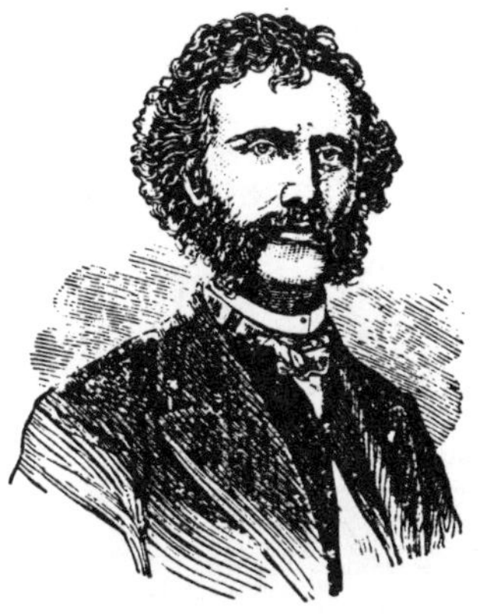

The great success I have met with, and the rapidly increasing demand for goods of my manufacture, is owing mainly to the superior quality of hair which I import exclusively for my trade, and the superior workmanship in their manufacture.

WIGS! WIGS! WIGS! WIGS!

I have the largest assortment of Wigs in the United States, and manufacture to order any and every style.

GENTS' WIGS AND TOUPEES,

Ventilated on human hair gauze or silk seams. Weft Wigs and Toupees, with or without seams, of straight or natural curly hair.

LADIES' WIGS,

Short or long glossy hair, straight, natural curly or frizzed. Also Fronts and Bandeaux.

DIRECTIONS FOR MEASURING THE HEAD FOR A WIG:

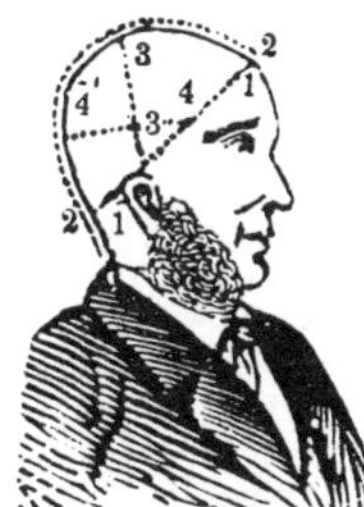

DIRECTIONS FOR MEASURING FOR TOUPEE OR SCRATCH:

No. 1.— The circumference of the head.

No. 2.—From the forehead to the nape.

No. 3.—From ear to ear, over the top of the head.

No. 4.—From temple to temple, round back of the head.

To measure for Toupee or Scratch, cut a piece of paper the exact size and shape of bald spot. Mark the crown and parting.

Send your orders according to the above directions, and I will warrant a fit.

I offer to the public the largest assortment of SWITCHES, CURLS, BRAIDS and FRIZZETTES, to be found in any establishment in America, and

DEFY COMPETITION IN QUALITY AND PRICE.

TAT-SI-O-KA-MA;

OR,

Mark Campbell's Japanese Hair Dye,

THE ONLY BROWN DYE IN THE WORLD.

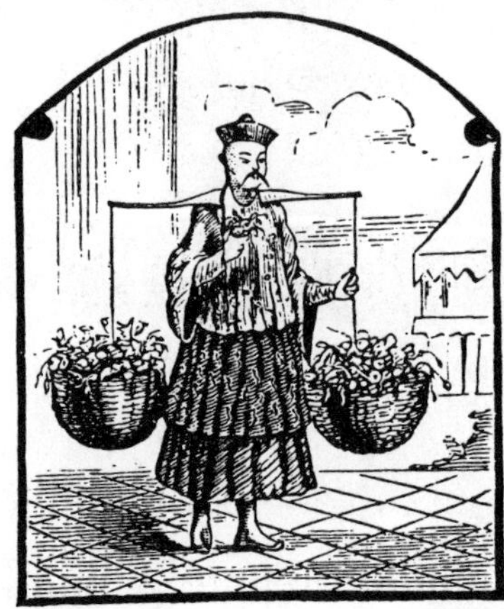

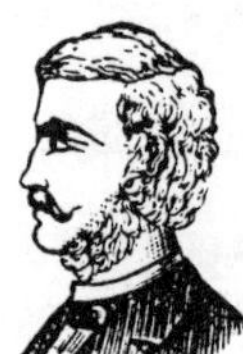

BEFORE USING.

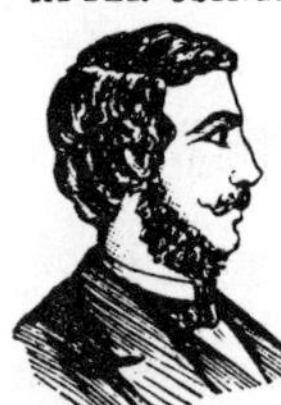

AFTER USING.

M. CAMPBELL'S JAPANESE BROWN HAIR DYE,

For Restoring the Hair to its Natural Color.

This wonderful Preparation needs only to be used to be appreciated. It is free from those objections that accompany preparations compounded from minerals, which have been offered to the pnblic in

Imitation of Brown Hair Dye.

It will restore the natural color of the Hair with but two or three applications. It is a common practice with compounders, when presenting an article to the public, to advertise an array of testimonials purporting to be from distinguished persons; but I prefer to rest the success of the Dye strictly upon its efficacious merit,

Knowing It Will Do All that is Claimed.

Warranted no Lac Sulphur, no Sugar of Lead.

Sold by all the principal Druggists in this country, and prepared by M. CAMPBELL, New York and Chicago.

ROBARE'S AUREOLINE;

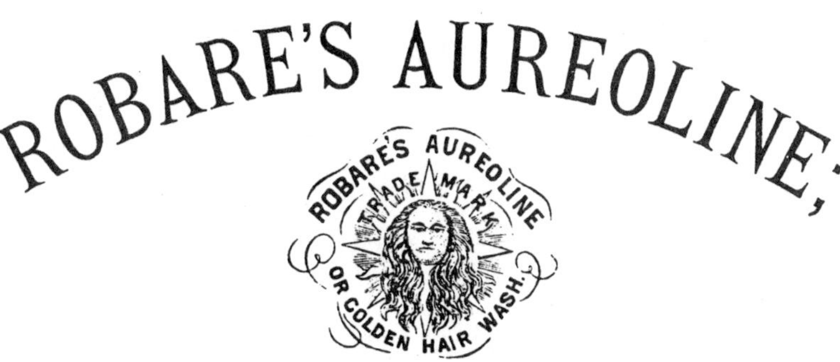

Or, Golden Hair Wash.

THIS PREPARATION, free from all objectionable qualities, has been discovered by the proprietor, after many experiments and much labor. By its use, after a few applications, the Hair gradually acquires that beautiful Sunny Hue, or Golden Color, so universally sought after and admired.

THE "AUREOLINE,"

From the harmless nature of the ingredients which enter into its composition, may be used without fear, even by the most timid. By its mild stimulating action the growth of the hair is promoted, and, from its strengthening qualities, any tendency to falling off is arrested.

DIRECTIONS FOR USE.

By means of a soft brush, distribute the AUREOLINE uniformly through the hair, in the same manner as would be adopted with an ordinary hair wash. Its application may be continued daily until the desired tint is obtained. In those cases where much grease has been employed, it is advisable to wash the hair previously with a weak solution of soda and water.

MANUFACTURED ONLY BY J. ROBARE, LONDON.

Wholesale and Retail Agent:

M. CAMPBELL, CHICAGO.

CAMPBELL'S GOLDEN TONIC.

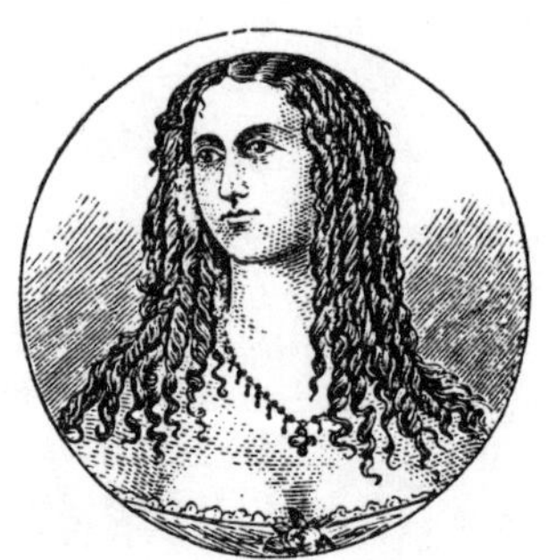

Campbell's Golden Tonic

FOR

RESTORING THE COLOR AND GROWTH OF THE HAIR.

IT IS A PREVENTIVE

AND

SURE CURE FOR BALDNESS,

Cleansing the Scalp of Dandruff and all Impurities, Invigorating the Roots of the Hair, giving it Life, Health and its Natural Color; also

CURES HEADACHE WITH MAGICAL EFFECT.

Hundreds of cases where the Hair was dropping, and Baldness seemed inevitable, have been effectually cured by the use of the Golden Tonic.

PREPARED ONLY BY

M. CAMPBELL.

SOLD BY ALL THE PRINCIPAL DRUGGISTS IN THIS COUNTRY.

PRICE, $1.00 PER BOTTLE.